THE HERBALIST
YOUR HEALING JOURNEY

by Jesse Wolf Hardin

Foreword by Mason Hutchison
–HerbRally–

Plant Healer Publications & Events
PlantHealer.org
(C) 2023 – Plant Healer Magazine LLC

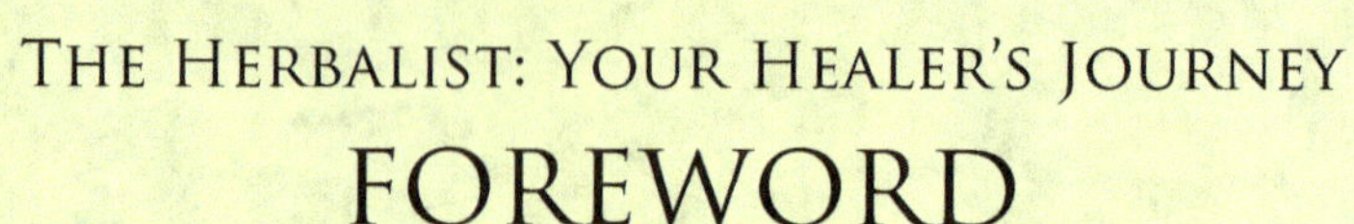

FOREWORD

by Mason Hutchison

I've been digital pen pals with Wolf for over a decade now. He writes some of my favorite emails I get in my inbox, full of stories, insight, life updates, wisecracks and the occasional unabashed vulgarity, and he always genuinely asks how I'm doing.

Then he emailed me with an idea: He wanted to create videos encapsulating some of the healing lessons he's learned over the course of his life, and offered to share them through the HerbRally YouTube channel. Understandably, as a self-identified luddite he wasn't stoked on the idea of creating a brand new social media account to share his message. I was so moved that Wolf wanted to share his message with the HerbRally audience, I may have shed a tear.

Thus, I enthusiastically wrote back verbatim: "To say I'm excited at the prospect of doing this is an *understatement!*" …and so *The Plant Healer's Path* series was born. Wolf began recording these five to twenty minutes long episodes and emailing them to me almost immediately. That's one thing I love about him — not only does he have ideas, but then he takes action. And in true Wolf fashion, he felt driven to turn it into a book. For one thing, he's a writer first. And for another, he understands that we all learn in different ways and didn't want to exclude his avid readers. That's what you have in your hands now, the text version of the first year's episodes.

Get ready to be inspired, uplifted, and empowered to be the very best healer you can be, and a misfit health provider without reservation.

I am excited for the herbal community and the world at large to benefit from the teachings of *The Plant Healer's Path* for generations to come.

—Mason Hutchison
The HerbRally Schoolhouse,
YouTube, Podcast & Event Directory
HerbRally.com

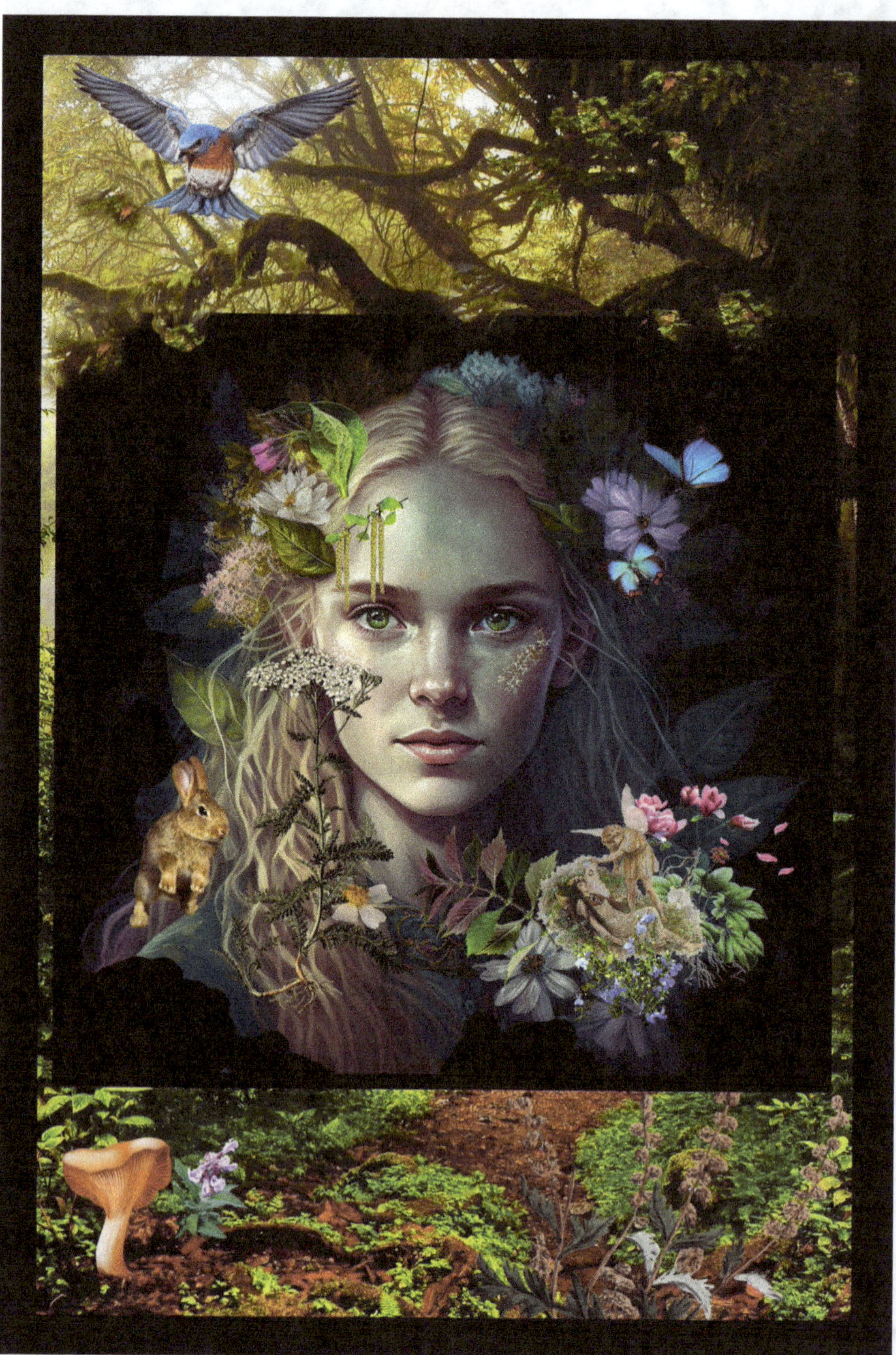

THE HERBALIST
—YOUR HEALER'S JOURNEY—

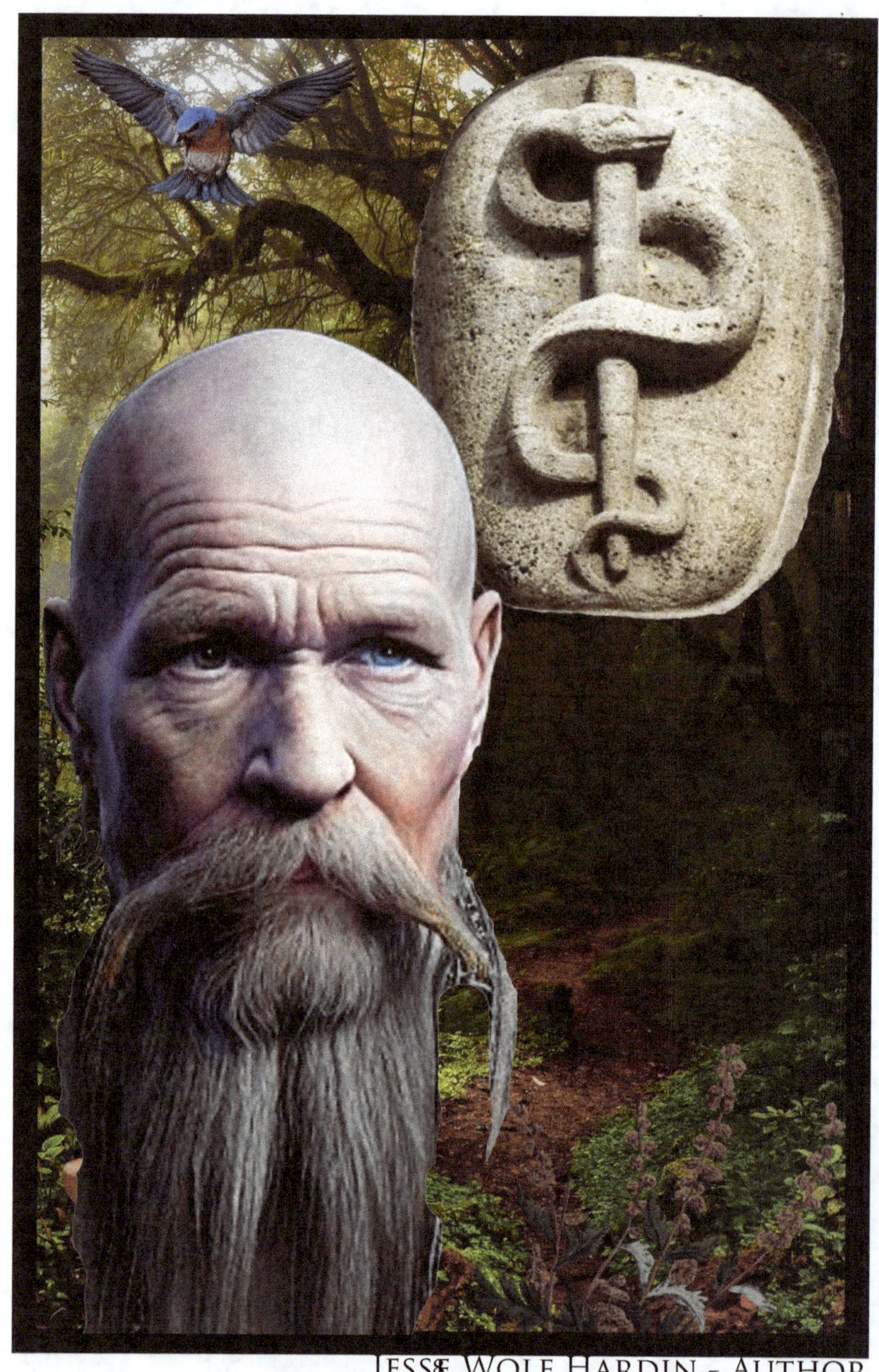

Jesse Wolf Hardin - Author

INTRODUCTION

by Jesse Wolf Hardin

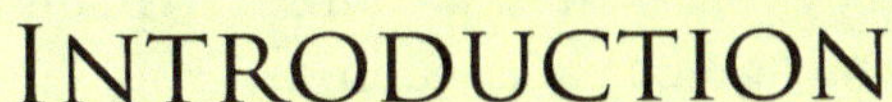

Welcome to the pages of another wolfen tome, 29 more catalytic chapters for all you purveyors of plants and virtual alchemists of healing.

Over the years we've produced dozens of compilation books for practitioners, filled with quite lengthy sections going into great depth about things like specific health conditions and materia medica, and in most cases pulled directly from illustrated issues of Plant Healer Quarterly magazine… but not so the following.

Chapters of *The Herbalist: Your Healer's Journey* are instead transcribed from the video series I've been creating for HerbRally, and therefore you'll find that each gets rather quickly to its promised point — non-typically in an unbridled conversational tone, with little extraneous padding and admittedly scant filters.

This is a faster tempo, no-brakes version of my characteristic teachings, described somewhat generously by associates as "wildling counsel," "plant hearted sermons," and "green cheerleading." You'll note that my focus is on providing practical tips and important information for anyone either practicing or just starting in herbalism and other healing modalities, from the various skills and steps needed to dealing with money, vital self-care, and how to determine your optimal personal specialty, role and niche in this field — but yes, this is as much as anything a compendium of hopeful inspiration and relentless encouragements! It's the "you and your healing work matters" book, the "magic is alive," "it's ok to be different," "you can do it" and "ain't it wondrous" book!

And wonder-filled indeed, is the essential Plant Healer mission of helping this planet, our diverse cultures, these lands and people, helping to heal from disease and disharmony and debility, helping contribute to wholeness in times of separation, polarization, and isolation. Wonderful is the incredible intensity of your empathy and caring, your determination to assist, and the poetic grace and utter delight you bring to your personalized version of our great and needed work. And wonderful, too, the plants that you work with, learn from, and share the blessings of. In every herbal root and leaf — as in every one of *you* — I see miracles of mending, and evocations of evolving beauty and meaning and purpose.

I poured all my heart and experience into this volume, and just as you so lovingly serve others *I dearly hope that it serves you well.*

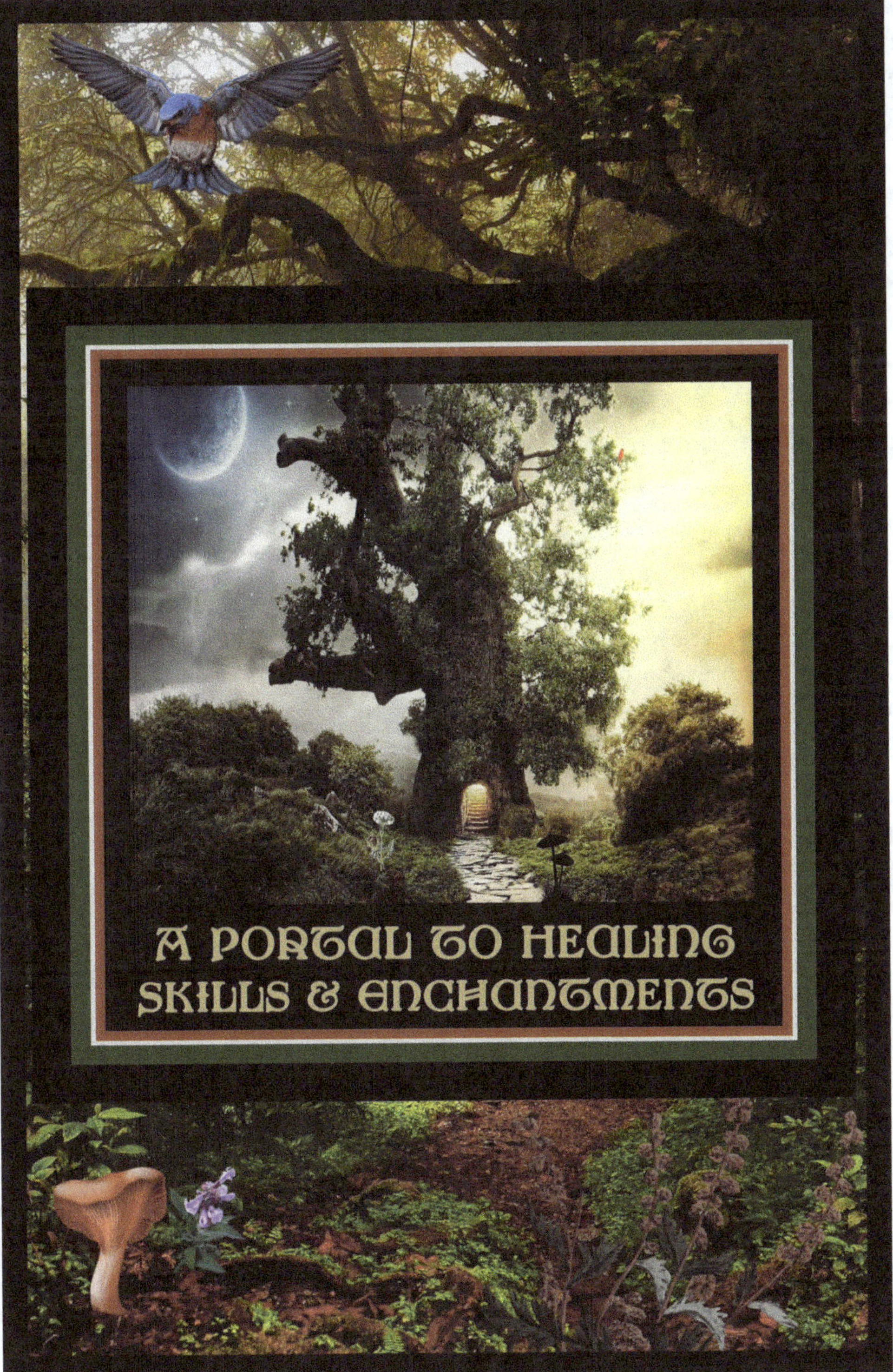
A PORTAL TO HEALING
SKILLS & ENCHANTMENTS

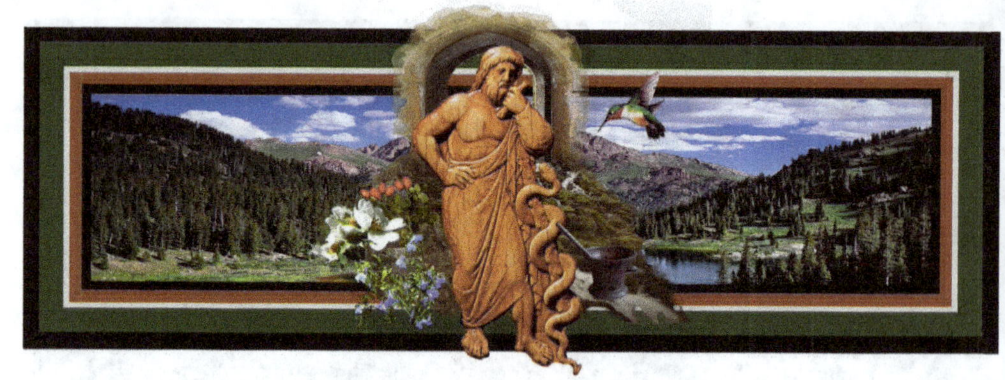

THE PORTAL
ENTRANCE TO THE WONDERMENTS OF LIFE, PURPOSE & HEALING

Something awaits you, at this very moment, and no matter where the hell you might be. It beckons from the shadow-mottled periphery of your daily life, from those thorn lined borderlands where the conscious and the unconscious, the familiar and the unknown meet.

Try as you might to ignore them, you cannot help but hear the wind-like whisperings of the improbable but possible — gesturing from just beyond the range of normal human sight. Step away even briefly from the narrow path of your assumptions and your routines, and it will almost certainly reveal itself, like a misty magical doorway into an enchanted forest through which you must intrepidly pass in order to experience the fullest expression of what it means to be your authentic self, living a life of deep meaning, fulfilling your personal special purpose. We enter, if we will, through the vehicle of our childlike curiosity and seeker's wonderment, through the hollow of an ancient tree, the suggestions of a swaying flower, or an herb's certain medicine.

For us, plants are not simply beautiful landscapes, nutritious meals or even curative herbs, so much as gestures to come outside, or to look closer at even the dried herbs in the jars on our shelves. They engage us with their smells and tastes, point to new realizations with their fabulous forms and actions, and capture our attentions away from the trivial and superficial with their motions, waving us forward to and through the portals again and again.

Every plant is itself an opening. Every part of every plant. Every aspect of every part. Every aspect's every effect... all are potential entrances to the very feelings that likely led us into the work of envisioning and healing in the first place. I can scarcely think of a research-minded phytotherapist who does not nearly trip over themselves upon discovery of a new medicinal species found growing in the area, or make sounds of satisfaction over a particularly positive case outcome... or bend over too far with their magnifying glass, getting closer and closer until tumbling forward into the wonder and oneness of this magical plant-infused natural world — a world of healing and wholeness.

It is to such portals we go to hear the earth's stories and heed its plaintive pleas, to be closest to the source and know the pleasures of its spell. And it is there, too, that we connect with the others of our kind and calling, an enchanted rendezvous where we co-create a reality informed by the medicine and mysteries within and around us. We can walk together out of the constrictive paradigm, out of the traps of assumption, certainty, sobriety and gravitas, and through and under the foliage curtaining each special portal.... reinhabiting our sensate bodies, filling our individual roles, reconnecting to our joy. We are the healers of what needs healing, bodies and minds, cultures and ecologies — collaborators in the awesome and the miraculous, determined inhabitants of satisfaction and bliss.

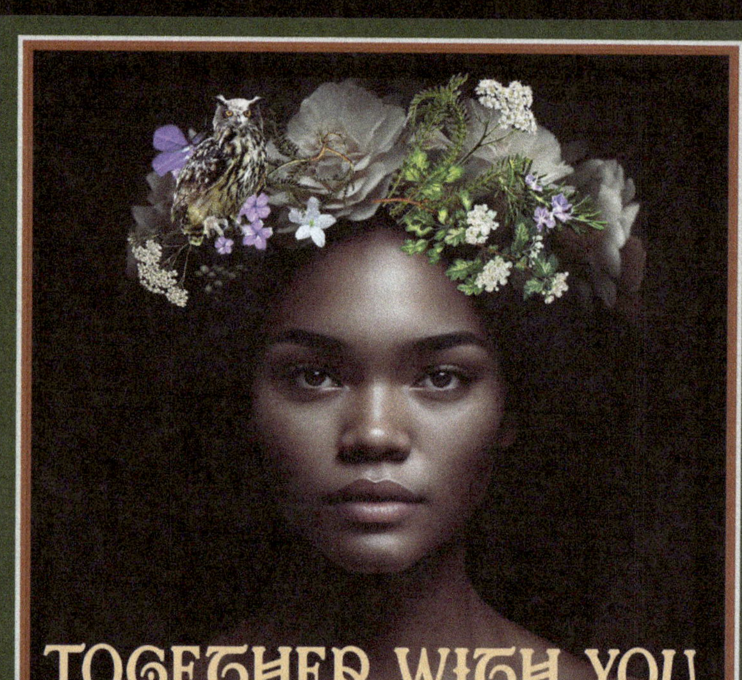

TOGETHER WITH YOU

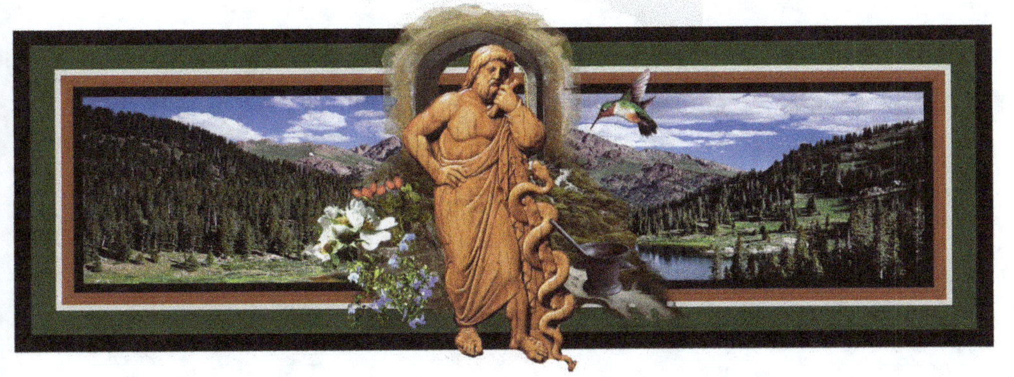

WHAT IS AN HERBALIST REALLY?

I've often been asked, "Just what does it mean to be —
or to become — an *herbalist*?"

According to the dictionary, an herbalist is simply:

1. a practitioner of herbalism or
2. a purveyor of medicinal herbs

As inclusive as this definition might be, calling oneself an "Herbalist" can still feel a mite pretentious or uncomfortable, wearing a mantle that you want to be sure fits you.

If you are new to plant medicine, you might wonder "What is it I have to learn and do in order to qualify?," while those with years or even decades in this field can sometimes question if we truly know enough, if we have done enough or are "good" enough.

There are qualifications and criteria for the title for sure, but they might not be what people usually think they are.

To begin with, being a genuine herbalist is *not* determined by:

• Whatever degrees you may have attained, as valuable as they might otherwise be.
• Any official designations, as hard as you may work to earn them.
• The number of clients you have seen, nor by the amount of money that you earn.
• Or whatever amount of recognition or fame that you might ever receive.

It helps to remember that some of the most effective herbalists of all time have been self taught, highly unofficial, and largely unknown outside of the local communities that they so graciously served.

They're qualified nonetheless, the genuine article, and their street cred is totally earned.

Being an herbalist is made real by just a few key things:

• First off, by your utter passion for herbs, and your desire and determination to help others.
• Secondly, by your growing knowledge and your personal experiences with medicinal plants and people's different health conditions.
• It's made real through the personal discoveries that you make, and the customized formulas you orchestrate.
• By putting however much knowledge you gain to actual use, helping clients or friends treat their issues.
• And finally, your Herbalist title is made real by the positive outcomes you assist with, and by the relief and gratitude showing on the faces of all those you help.

To be clear, an herbalist is essentially *anyone and everyone who knowledgeably and effectively uses plants to help support the natural healing processes.*

Don't get me wrong — you can always study to learn more than what you know now, as you well should. In the future you can integrate different traditions, as well as experiment and come up with new methods and techniques… but accept the fact, you are *already* an herbalist.

Your role doesn't await you down the line like some distant goal post, it's right now, this moment, putting your current knowledge and overwhelming obsession to work — improving lives naturally!

Let me give you just a few suggestions for how to roll:

- Start working regularly with a small number of herb species, and then expand.
- Try a new tincture, and pay attention to how it feels and acts.
- Don't just buy herbs, wildcraft — gathering wild healing herbs even in the city.
- Get some soil on your hands even if you don't have a yard for a garden, at least try growing some potted herbs inside.
- Understand the plants as beings with their own intrinsic value, their own needs, and their own right to lives of dignity.
- Share your accumulating knowledge, and especially your actual experiences, with those who might benefit, whether a family member, a paying client, or with a suffering checker as you're waiting in line with fellow shoppers.
- If you find yourself consumed with herbs daily, consider developing your passion into a service or business, open a shop or a place for consultation, try going online to sell the herbal products that you make, find a means to teach students, write about what you know and what you speculate about.
- Finally, enjoy! Enjoy the intimate, sensual rituals of handling, smelling, tasting, and providing plants' special medicines. Take some credit for your part in healing and bettering our precious world.

Believe me, *you got this!*

If you care enough about herbs and healing, no amount of self doubt, fear or hesitancy can prevent what will evolve into your lifetime relationship and walk with the plants — a journey of learning and doing: your Plant Healer's path.

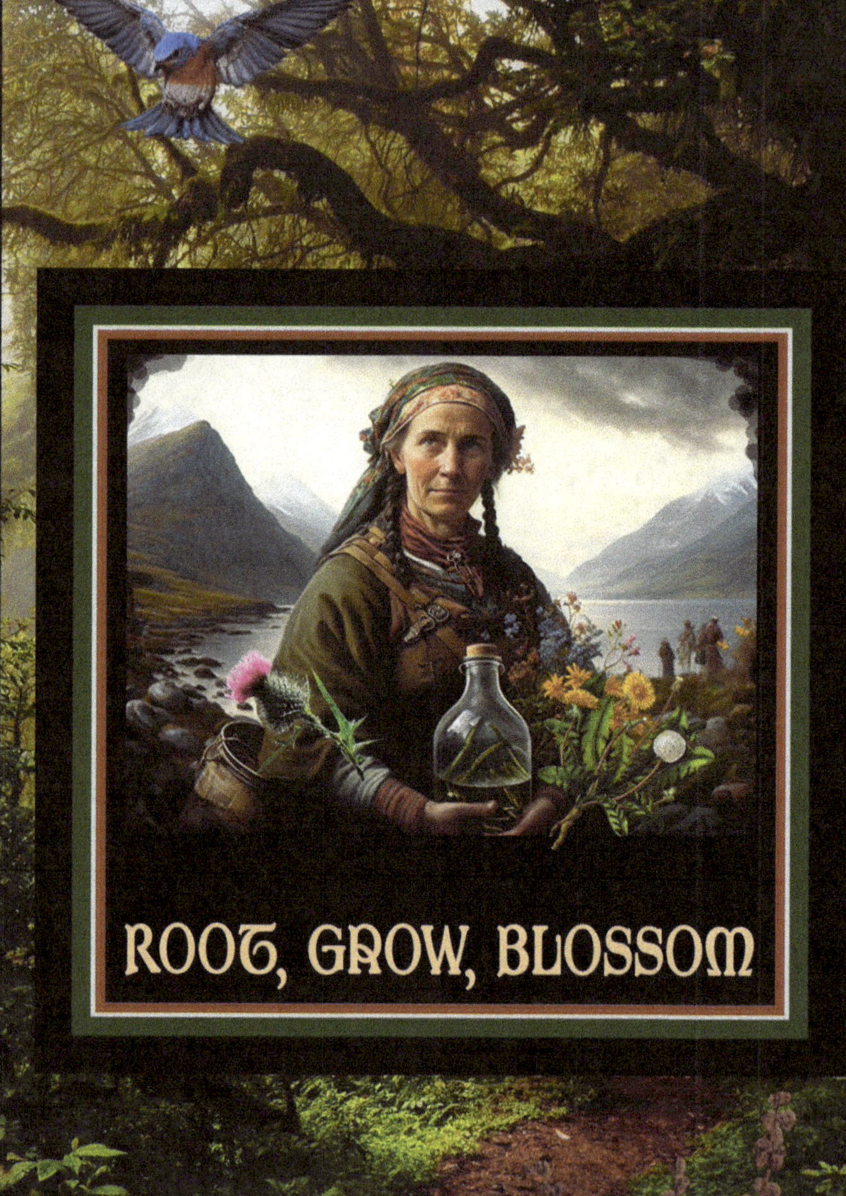
ROOT, GROW, BLOSSOM

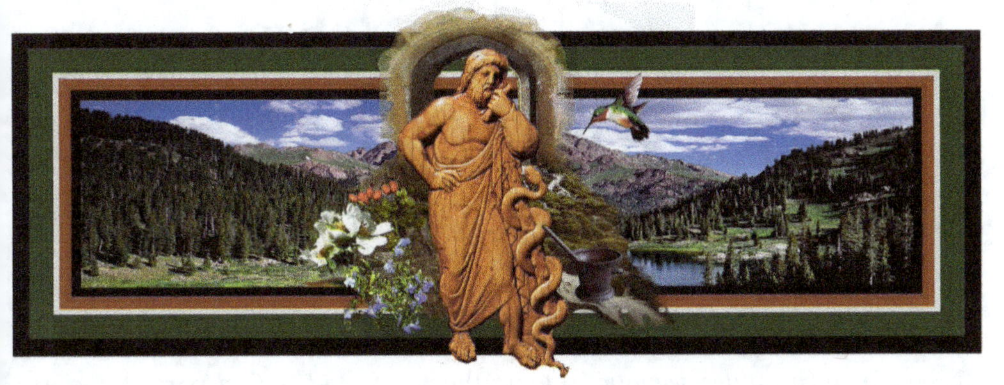

HERBSTORY

THE HISTORY, HEART & FUTURE
OF PLANT MEDICINE

The leaf-mulched soil underneath bushes and trees is sometimes referred to as their "story," as in "oak story." It is story, in that its composition tells us much about the nearby plant life and the soil's creation, about its fertility or lack thereof. So, too, does our beloved field of herbalism have an organic story, deeper than the various spins put out by uncritical zealots, critical industry spokespersons, and professional medical and herbal organizations. It the story of a living, inspirited planet expressing and fulfilling it itself through myriad evolving ways, including such purposeful extensions of itself as medicinally beneficial plants... and such as *us*, the responsive organs and agents of the organic whole that both scientists and cosmologists call "Gaia." We can see how fertile herbalism is today, where it is deficient.... as well as all the ways it is nutrient rich, as we subjectively run our hands through its humus and loam, reading to the best of our ability its evolving story.

This story begins with the plants themselves, and the carefully orchestrations of chemicals that benefit not only them but other elements of the ecosystem. And before the arrival of human kind, the animals were already making discoveries as to the medicinal benefits of some of the plants they ingest.

Tanzanian Chimpanzees were witnessed peeling the stems and eating the pith of the Vernonia plant (Bitter Leaf), a plant that has been found to exhibit anti-parasitic and anti-microbial properties. They were also seen to carefully roll the leaves of the Aspilia bush with the bristle side out before swallowing them whole, potentially effective in scouring their intestines of parasitic worms. Both species are part of the traditional materia medica of the Tanzanian people.

In other studies, it was found that the only baboons who ate the fruits of the Desert Date (*Balanites aegyptiaca*) were those infected with a parasitic worm carried by water snails. Other baboons, without the problem and need, showed little interest in the bitter fruits.

Bears have long been known to dig up various herbal bitters to aid digestion after eating a huge meal, earning a reputation among the tribal peoples of Asia and America as a "Medicine Animal," one that can lead us to the botanical treatments we need.

Medicine Men and Medicine Woman followed, learning the ways of the medicinal plants, and treating not only themselves but others in their families and villages. Thousands of years of herbal traditions follow, a period of denigration and repression, then a 20th Century revival.

Today we recognize two somewhat contradictory courses:

1. the isolation of components, the commodification of plant medicine, and attempts to win acceptance from the system through certification, and

2. a resurgence of folk traditions, herbal education for the everyday person, access to natural health care for the disenfranchised and impoverished, responsibility and personal empowerment in the face of commercial pressures, public attitudes, and repressive legislation.

We are at a historic crossroads, with one of our possible options being an always sober study, expression and practice, and with a second possible choice being an emotion-filled, sensual, playful, celebratory, liberatory, diligent but joyous herbalism that is everyday not just a blessing to others but also a reward to us.

We harken back to the earliest expressions of nature's health and healing, and we are a part of a lineage of caring, helping and healing that connects us to all who came before, and to every care giver and plant healer that will ever arise to help perform this ancient service. Together, in the now, we co-create a resurgent culture of healing. Herbalism will always exist in some form or another so long as there are people (or chimpanzees, or bears...) alive and helpful plants to be treasured and utilized... but the form it takes will to a large extent depend on us. We are called not just to learn some plant medicine and share it with others, but to develop a vision of the best of what can be... the work and pleasure so clearly meant for you.

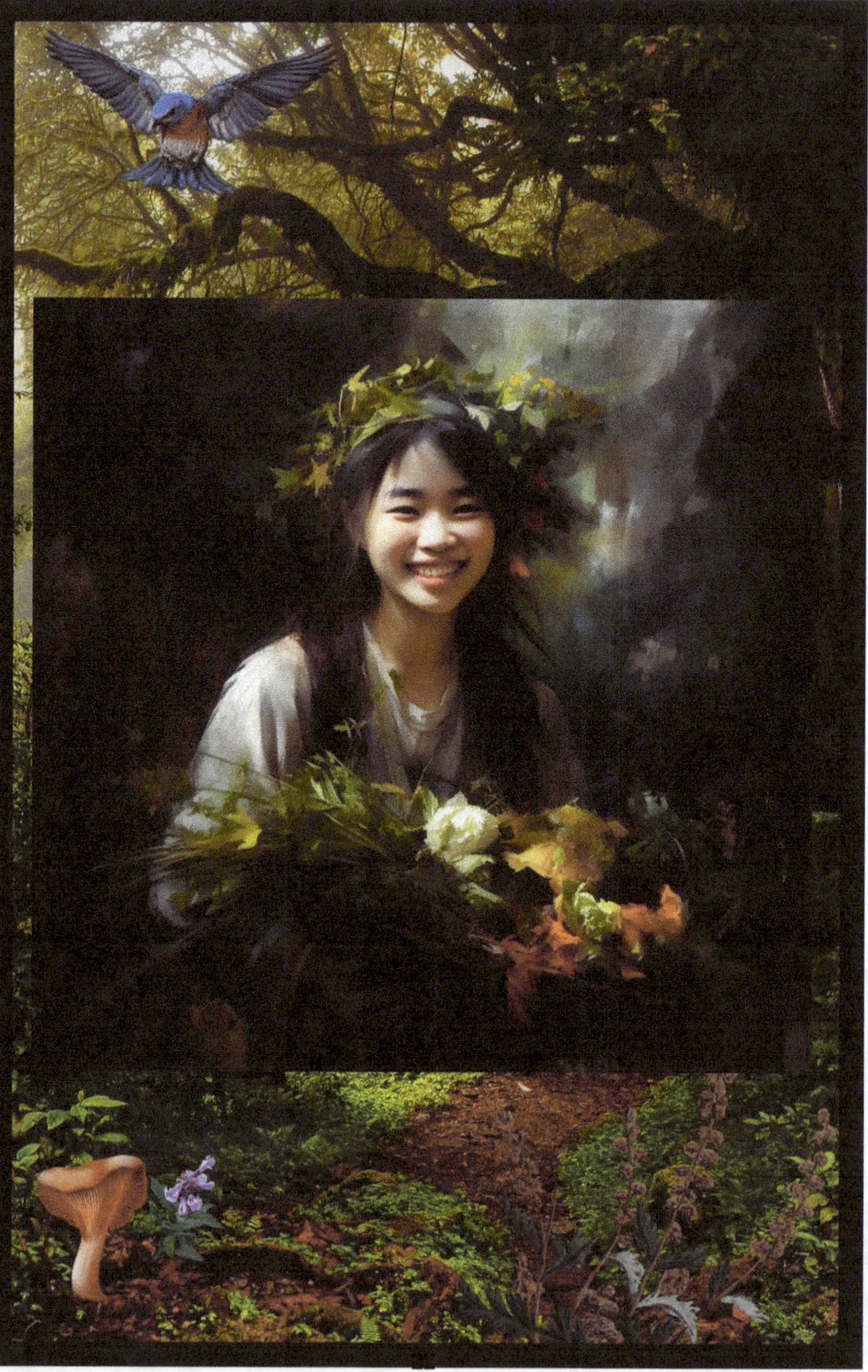

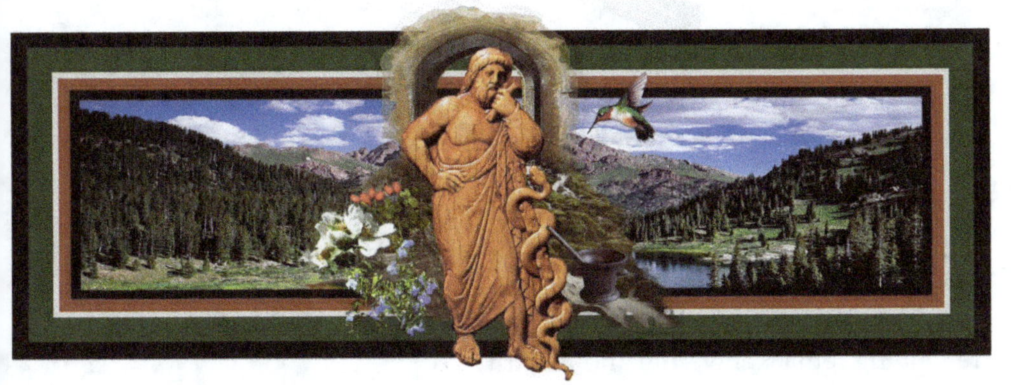

THE REAL MEANING
OF HEALTH & HEALING

My dictionary defines "Health" simply as an "absence of illness or injury". Now c'mon — how ridiculous is that? There are zillions of people without a specific illness or any obvious debility who are nonetheless far from any measure of what it means to be truly *well*.

Other ways to measure wellbeing should surely include:

- First of all, vitality, vigor, physical energy, and overall oomph

- Having mental clarity, responsiveness, motivation, and a degree of ability to deal with stress

- Functionality — with shit not just surviving or doing the bare minimum, but actually working well

- The relative strength of bone and muscle, the strength of different organ actions, and a strong immune response

- The presence of an effective microbiome, that community of bacteria needed for good digestion and nutrient assimilation

- And lastly, finding meaning in one's life, having a sense of purpose, hope for the future, and feelings of fulfillment

It's also inaccurate to think of healing as just the elimination of, or the reduction of, problematic symptoms. Such focus on symptoms can easily result in insufficient attention being given to underlying foundational causes — for example, the overlooking of degraded liver function or an autoimmune condition, failing to diagnose a vitamin B12 deficiency, or failing to take into account harmful lifestyle habits. Obviously someone might have zero symptoms and still have some mighty serious problems, or someone can have certain recurrent symptoms while in most ways remaining remarkably vital and healthy.

My definition of health is "wholeness," and thus the call to heal is to "help make whole." For the Plant Healer, the object is not simply to address symptoms, nor is it even to "cure" a condition, so much as it is to assist a "return to balance and wholeness" of people's bodies, minds and spirits, of our fractured societies, and of the entire natural world we arise from and depend upon.

Whenever a person or a thing is un-whole, there's an *imbalance* created – a dangerous tipping caused by essential weighty parts being either missing, excised, reduced, repressed or ignored. When someone or something is out of balance, they do not act out of their true natures or in ways that serve their aims and intentions. Imbalance can result in neglected needs or volatile reactions, inappropriate or untimely responses, the self sabotaging of our relationships and endeavors, and the undermining of our chances for satisfaction. Bodily systems are in the greatest danger when they've been knocked out of balance — whether by injuries or infection, introduced toxins or nutritional depletion. The same can be said when it comes to endangered ecosystems, or even mental and emotional health. And if we are seriously out of balance, it's going to be hard for us to even do the essential work of healing ourselves and others, and crazy hard to run forwards on our purposed paths without losing our way or even falling on our face.

Herbal tonics can have a balancing effect on our energies and bodily systems, herbal adaptogens like Ashwagandha can support internal equilibrium, particular vitamins and minerals can have a dramatic benefit. Reintroducing balance also requires the recognition and reintegration of what are often long-missing parts of the person, and elements from dietary nutrients to self acceptance, time in a forest, the heeding of a sidelined calling, and the following of our dreams. The regaining of balance is one of the keys means to re-becoming whole — and thus of *healing*.

We do our best work when we're active in consciously healing our own beings, our family and clients, and this living earth. We do our best when assisting the body's, the community's and the land's inherent ability and natural inclination to heal themselves — which is why the supportive actions of plant medicines are so very important.

We have the longest lasting effects when we take the time to determine the environmental, nutritional, personal and lifestyle imbalances that cause or worsen the many maladies we encounter, and when we recommend the kinds of changes most likely to help prevent further occurrences.

And irrespective of particular outcomes, the healer's work is deepened by paying attention to those valuable lessons that all maladies provide, deepened from the actual effects of different herbs. Deepened by any new insights into how bodies need to be cared for.   And deepened by a metaphysical reappraisal of what really, truly matters most in life.

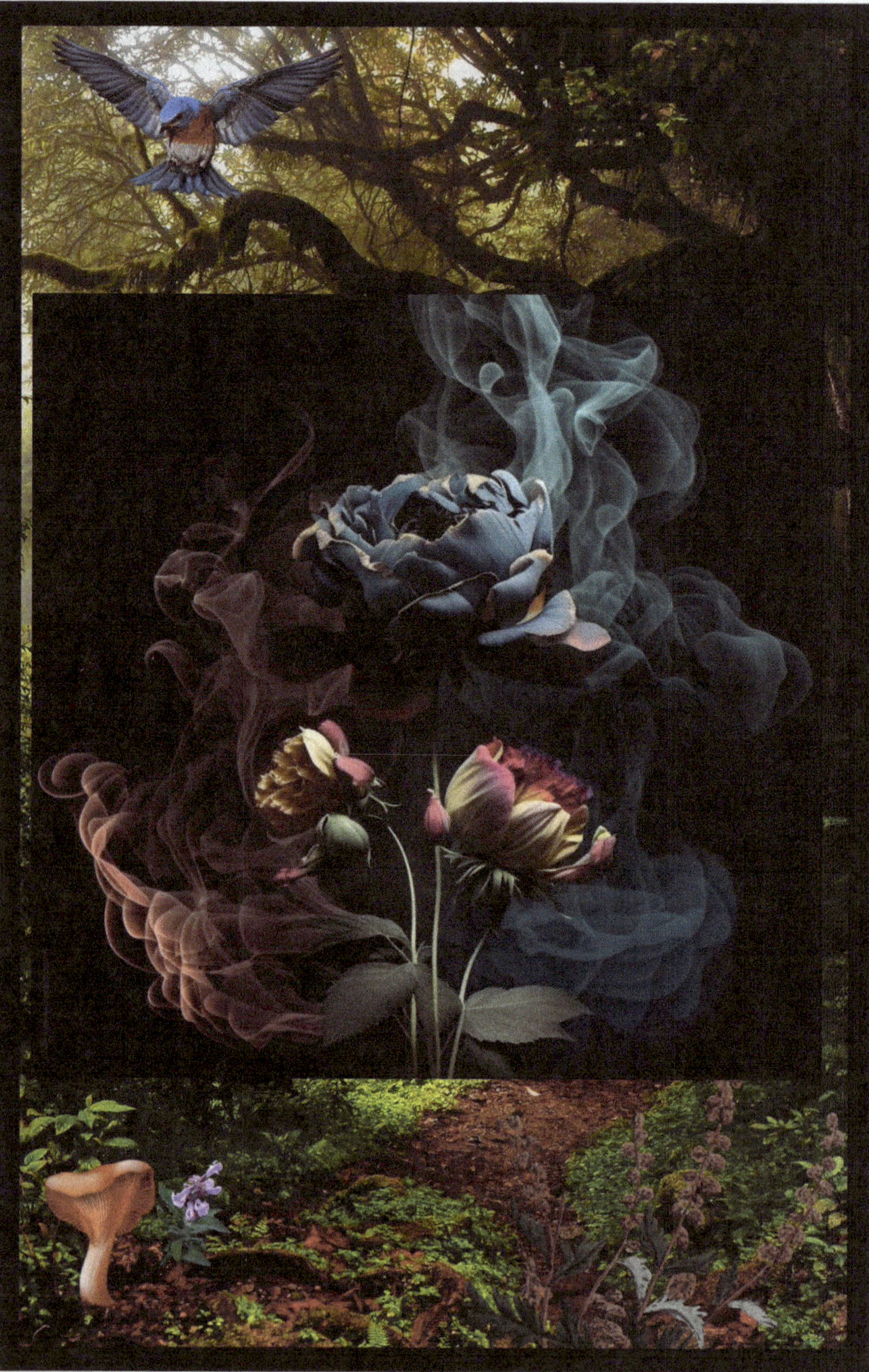

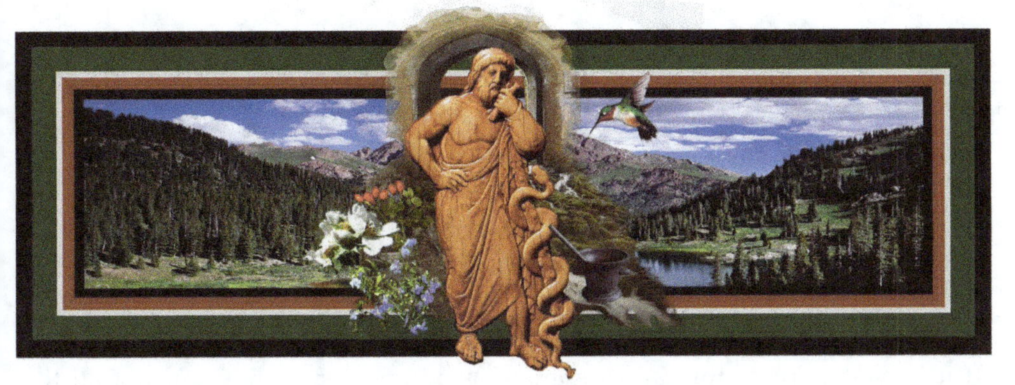

BEAUTY & THE PLANT

THE LOVELY IN OUR CARING
& PURPOSED LIVES

There was a period in my activist years when I spoke little of beauty, whispered like a soft wind, through stiffened lips like protective gates. As with my chef's knives or woodsman's axe, I never denied its existence or purpose, but kept it high in a drawer so no one could be hurt by its incautious wielding.   To the degree that I neglected to acknowledge the attractive, or to praise the lovely, such reticence grew out of inescapable images of young girls crying because their beauty did not conform to an overly symmetrical and undernourished ideal, being told that my artwork is a foolish and counterrevolutionary indulgence when there is so much ugliness to transmute and evil to confront. Later, I often heard how beauty was a construct of the dominant paradigm, an artificial concept imposed upon the people by an elite concerned with separating and controlling us, furthering division, hierarchy and classism.   To say that something or someone is beautiful, I was told, is to make clear that we think other things are less pretty, that other people are not as comely or valuable.

Now the word "beauty" rises often, like blossoms released underwater by free spirited mermaid gardeners, and breaking the surface one after the other. As with rain sprouted seeds after a drought, there is no way to hold back the words of praise and adoration so long unwatered.

These eruptions of adoration and amazement need not pad their steps as they make their way through ears and hearts, nor recoil in fear of the shame faced pillory, for they emerge as a forgotten language, speaking in and to a different society, in a different if parallel time. It is here in this otherly context that beauty describes a loveliness apart from the stereotyping, marginalization, and dissing, here that this word glows and shimmers like gifted flowers.

If it is neglectful or hurtful to name one thing as appealing but not all the rest, it's an even greater harm to silence our amazement and approbation, to withhold our subjective, naturally felt attraction and adoration. If we are drawn to the purple preciousness of a lone Sweet Violet, surrounded by a host of eager yellow Strawflowers or subtle Oats, it is not to disparage common blossomings, nor to slight their sepia-toned neighbors with their rustling seed heads – it is, instead to voice a very personal affection and delight, that God or the Gods are welcome to overhear, and that future generations are invited to read. And it is through our expressed praise, excitement, and connection, that other people may be inspired to find and sing out about those things in their lives and work, homes and regions, which beckon and pleasure them most.

Expressions of beauty – the *very potential* for beauty – lies in all things like a winged seed, like a sparkle when an object or being is turned just the right way, or a previously unheard tone emanating from deep within.

Everyone who views or hears it, does so at a slightly different angle, from a particular perspective determined by not just orientation but by their cultures and experiences, traumas, delights, and needs. It is thus that not all agree on what is most beautiful, even when we agree that there are elements of beauty in everything… and so should it be, for it is not an agreement in danger of becoming fad or convention, it is a measure and description of ourselves as much as of that which we've beheld.

What we consider attractive or repellent is subjective: They are subject to our abilities to notice or not, our discernment and selection or our overlooking and dismissal. Likewise, we are subject to their appearance and effects.

This not to say that there is no seemingly incontrovertible ugliness in the world, things that resound like the utterly distasteful ingredients of a recipe for disquiet and disease, so repugnant as to be avoided by most people, scrutinized in fable, and vilified in the diverse customs of ice dwellers, rainforest residents, isolated towns and crowded metropolises alike. As with beauty, examples abound: the guarded or self assured expressions of prevaricators, most actions that frighten children, oil-soaked beaches after a spill, miles of too-straight colorless template buildings and the wince worthy neon colors sometimes used to dress them up.

So too, there is beauty that only those of a certain ilk recognize, like old friends or reunited family, like finding home in a way and place you have never before seen. If it is examples you want, let us consider the beauteous shining faces of babies and babblers to the gorgeousness of one's lover. And the hopeful glinty sunrises and mesmerizing rose and gold sunsets to those ensconced too long indoors and grateful for those eternal seconds outside. And flower blossoms – memory-baiting blood-red Roses, tear-jerking Lavender, and tiny Anenomes the color of many a newborn's eyes. Flowers whispering "look at me" from distant fields. Flowers dried and strung into the wreaths of women gazing out their windows, with crazy amounts of embroidery on their sunlit peasant blouses. Flowers gingerly left on doorsteps by bashful suitors. Flowers as intimates, unfurling their flavors in crystal teapots, hung in careful bundles from the rafters of community healers, decocted and infused into bottles that are themselves beautiful.

I feel like a barefoot explorer of the utterly exotic found within the ever so familiar, an enraptured bard setting my ceaseless admiration to a danceable beat. As such, I find beauty in your Plant Healer's commitment, in the way you not just gently but gracefully place a hand upon a sore belly to offer comfort while making your assessment, in your waterfall laughter when you discover a new and helpful species of herb, in your eyes when you are enamored, excited, entranced, or invigorated by the elements and actions of your work. I can barely look away from the arrangements of bottled herbs on your pantry shelf, and see beauty in things so simple and precious as the the lay of the herbalist's knife on your plant strewn table.

Who would we most want to entrust our wellbeing to? The answer is that most naturally, hopefully, and pleasurably, it would be those caregivers inspired by a compassionate desire to provide relief and contribute to that mysterious choreography we call vitality, those informed by a shameless connection to beauteous nature and personal experience, they who are irretrievably obsessed with the power, dignity, and beauty of the healing plants themselves.

If there be elves and faeries, and if they still on rare occasion enjoy the interests and applaud the actions of humans, then surely they do so for those herbalists who delight in pretty things, and who chance their heart to the overly beautiful and manifestly meaningful.

The blandness of concrete and asphalt, calls for the noticing of the colors of a porch flower-box, an appreciation for the green of a lawn and the rainbow arc of sunbeams dancing on a sprinkler's spray. The ugliness of endless hateful wars, needs the contrast of compassionate deeds and gorgeous sunrises. The ill need not just the dispiriting awareness of their plight or pain, but an awareness of the beauty in a caregiver's smile, in words of kindness, in the lifting and swaying of one's own hair when a hospital rule is broken and a window opened. Just the knowledge of highly depressing events can lead to unhealthiness and decline, which is why we do well to dance with the fancies of death, sing in the face of fear, encourage humor within the twists and convolutions, notice the light that shares stage with the dark, and find beauty in the substance and evocation of attendant life, and magic, and love. Atop a sadly melting glacier, one can dry their eyes and look deep into its remaining frozen depths, and still be lifted and blessed by its crystalline bubbles and amazing aqua blue sheen.

But beauty is seldom frozen or still, it changes with its own cycles of melt and rebuild. It tumbles out in brilliant notes from plaintive violins, bouncing bass dance beats, the lungs of culture changing songsters and the throats of the the shameless, the celebratory, the bereaved. It tumbles like light through an apothecary's bottles, remade and re-toned by their cobalt curves and amber recesses, like the rainbow infused drops of mystic river spray, like the tumbling laughter of wise fools and the crazily in love.

I leave it to others to proclaim that beauty is as ephemeral as a seldom visiting ghost, as temporary as a beeswax candle which everyone knows burns much faster than petroleum paraffin. If I am to shout anything to the winds and those who ride them, it would be this: That the Jay birds outside my window are as blue the water of our dreams, are beautiful from the moment they are visible, wet-feathered with pink patches of dinosauric skin and a spiky hairdo usually associated with bespectacled old men. They are astonishingly pretty as they draw sharp angles in the sky outside our cabin, and when posturing like talkative suitors atop the branches of the Junipers and Pines and Piñons. And they're beautiful to me, even when perished and fallen to the earth, hollowed out and feathers unkempt, quieter than church, quieter than those moments after a lover tells us something impossible to respond to, impossible to hear. And if I myself were thus struck down, I would not want so much to have words spoken about my dogged insistence or myriad accomplishments, so much as folk noting that I had found things to be fascinating, and meaningful… and pretty. It would be recognized that in a world with its share of disease, I served wellness, and that in a time of great distractions and unpleasantries I found and gave myself to the lovely.

When we say something is "beautiful to me," we speak not of a beauty that is ours alone to own, not a secret tryst hidden from judgy eyes and therefore unbeknownst to the world, but rather, openly and credited, as in a "gift to me."

So, too, can it be a gift to you.

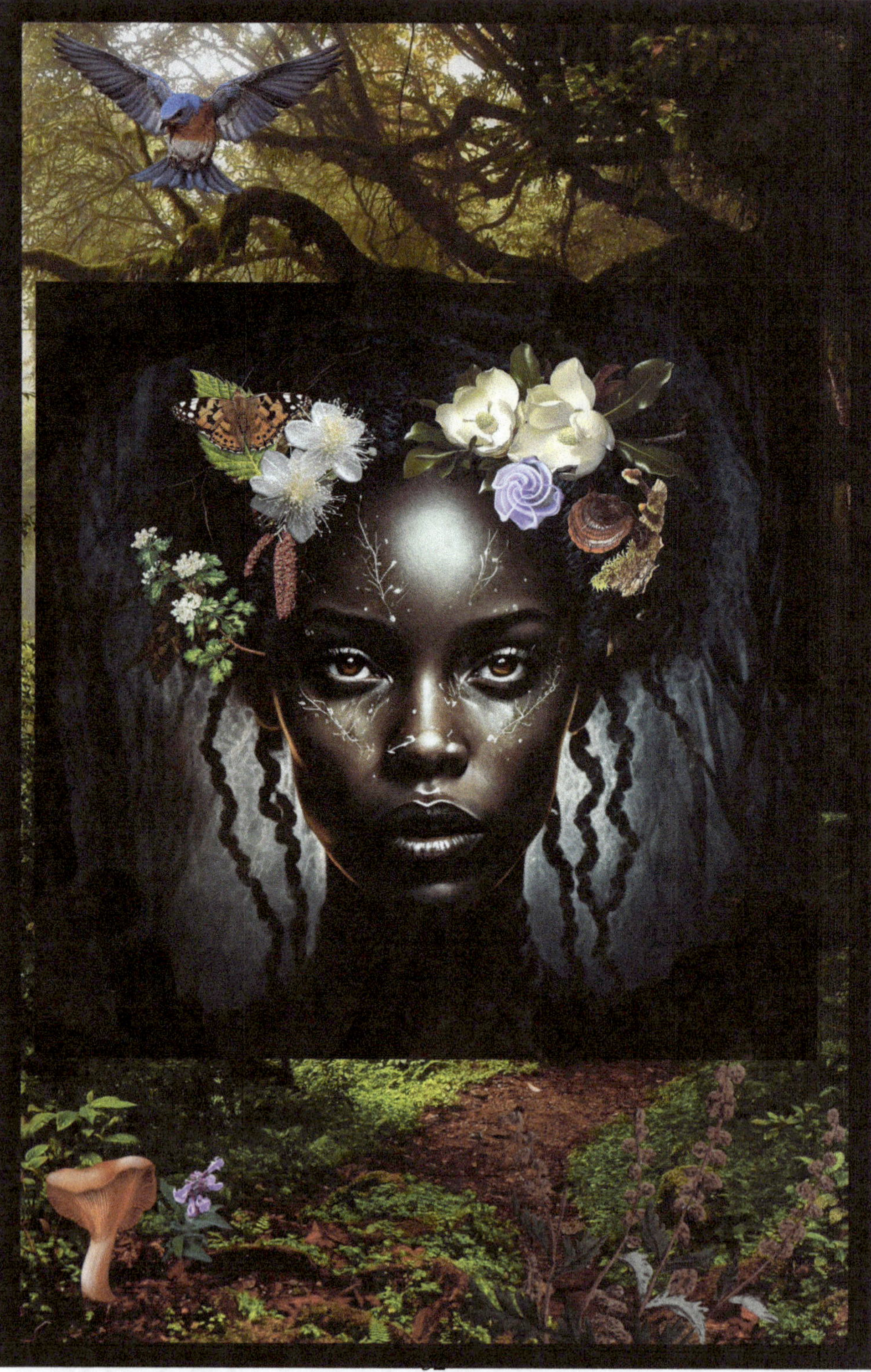

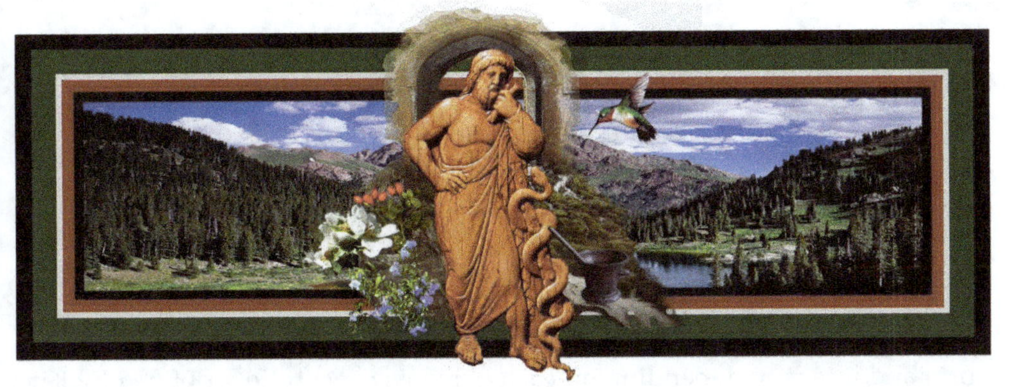

10 Things to Know
to be The Best Herbalist You Can Be

You can help people feel better and avoid harmful drugs, with really only the most rudimentary skills and knowledge. But believe me — there are definitely certain things to know in order to become *the very best herbalist that you can be.*

In my books *The Practice of Herbalism* and *The Plant Healer's Path*, I go into considerable detail about some of things you might want to think about learning, whether that involves your reading, apprenticing, or attending a school or online classes. Here are 10 of the most important:

#1: Herbal Actions & Attributions

As you know, herbalism is the study and use of medicinal herbs, perhaps most important being a deepening understanding of what conditions or issues each plant species is known to be used for, and learning what their specific actions and effects are on bodily systems and processes.

#2: Pathology & Diagnostics

Knowledge about plant medicines is foundational, but so is the study of the conditions, illnesses, symptoms and presentations that we're called upon to treat. Your ability to recognize problems and patterns are what make it possible for you to effectively address any issues causing imbalanced, debilities, and pain.

#3: Physiology & Anatomy

When addressing illnesses or injuries, you'd be right thinking it's important to know a little basic physiology and anatomy, meaning the locations and functions of bodily parts and organs.

#4: Constitutions & Energetics

The effects that active ingredients in medicinal herbs have on people vary in form and intensity depending on each person's constitution, defined by Kiva Rose as "our native/intrinsic and learned/adaptive patterns of personality and body traits." An understanding of constitutional models is a way of fine tuning a healing approach or herbal regimen to diverse individuals. We similarly tune-in to the plant medicines themselves, when we learn to credibly practice herbal energetics — using the human senses, especially taste and smell, to determine the likely properties and actions of even those herbs we are totally unfamiliar with.

#5: Medicine Making

Many herbs need to be processed, such as tinctured in alcohol or made into a topical balm, in order for their active ingredients to be bioavailable. This means we have to either purchase them from product sellers or else learn how to make them ourselves. Often your homemade medicines can be just as effective, or even more effective, than what you can buy, and this way you can custom tweak blends and compounds to suit an exact purpose or the needs and constitution of a particular person.

#6: Botany & Plant Identification

The way to be certain what plants we are working with, it to key them out ourselves, identifying them through their parts and shapes. Botany also seeks to explain each herb's physiology, its physical and chemical processes.

#7: Wildcrafting & Cultivation

As fresh and quality as some purchased herbs can be, it is often freshly harvested or wildcrafted plants prove the strongest. Gardening and foraging are both affordable means of procurement, and can be sustainable when done consciously and carefully.

Both growing and gathering in the wild can lead us into deeper connection to the plants themselves, interacting with them while they are still growing, thriving, and communicating. I suggest becoming intimate with the wild and feral medicinals growing even in the cities, and doing at least a little growing in indoor containers if not a full-on garden.

#8: Lifestyle & Nutrition

Physical conditions can seldom be fully addressed using herbs or drugs alone. Even the most effective plants cannot be expected to "cure" problems, arrest chronic imbalances or make up for deficiencies. Herbs are most helpful in concert with lifestyle changes, such as quitting or taking a break from an unhealthy relationship or a stressful job, getting better exercise, and especially improved nutrition. An herbalist who takes the time to evaluate the latest nutritional research, and who pays close attention to the effects of different foods on various constitutions and conditions, can usually be more helpful than someone using a strictly botanical approach.

#9: Counseling & Psychology

Herbalists are not in the job of giving counsel, and you would need to be licensed before offering legal "therapy," and yet it can be crucial for clients to have help with adjusting their perceptions and their unhealthy emotional patterns if they are to get well and stay well.

#10: Existing, Historic, & Traditional Forms of Herbal Practice:

Finally, nothing human exists outside of the context of human culture, and that's true for herbalism and healing in general. Cultures and histories help to inform, color and distinguish, including different ways of knowing and practicing plant medicine. We do well to study diverse traditional practices, different cultural perspectives, and the different herbs and methods used by different peoples in different places on the globe. Traditional Chinese Medicine, Ayurveda, African and Slavic folk healing, the insights of the indigenous peoples of South and North America, just to name a few.

We – and our contributions to the world – exist on a continuum of mentors and discoveries. We're each a part of a recurring blossoming of earth-informed healing, a lineage in which we serve as links connecting the herbalism and herbalists of the past to the plant medicine and the plant healers of the future!

We can accumulate all this valuable knowledge by reading specialized books on these fields and topics, such as those available through the Plant Healer Online Bookstore, by enrolling in physical or online herb schools, or by attending herbal education gatherings. Practical herbalist skills can also be learned this way, although the most instructive teachers of technique and application are your personal experiences. Nothing can take the place of actually working with the plants, and actually helping a wide range of people in need. Insights can come at any time, yet the longer one has been doing something, the more *able* we'll become.

Just remember — that all knowledge is most effective when combined with awakened physical senses, heightened awareness and practiced observation, developed discernment and incisive critical thinking, nonlinear thinking and intuition, synergy and reflection, passion, application, and action.

These are some of the things that can deepen, accelerate and equip you on our Plant Healer's Path — helping us become the very best, most effective herbalists that we can possibly be.

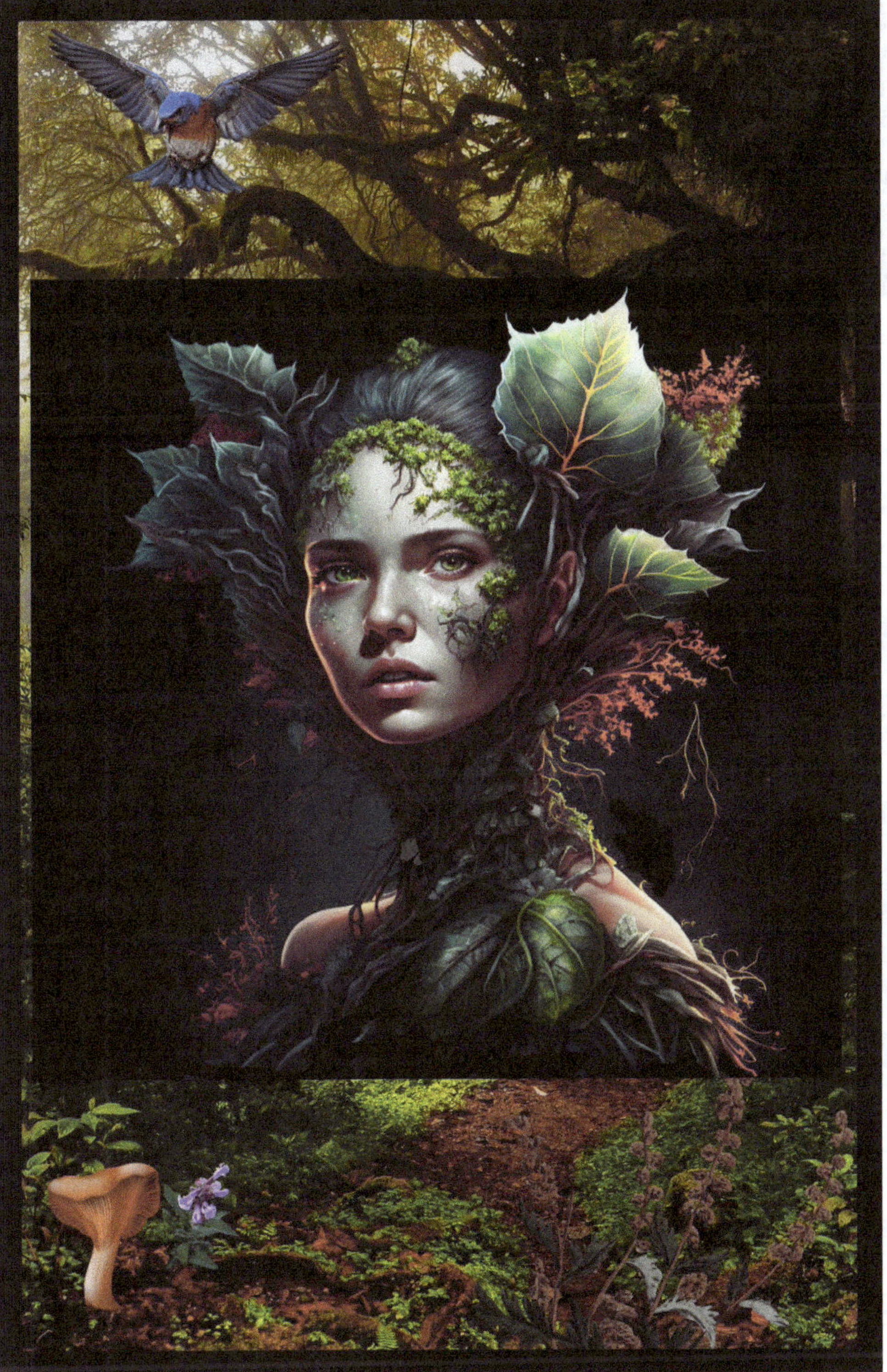

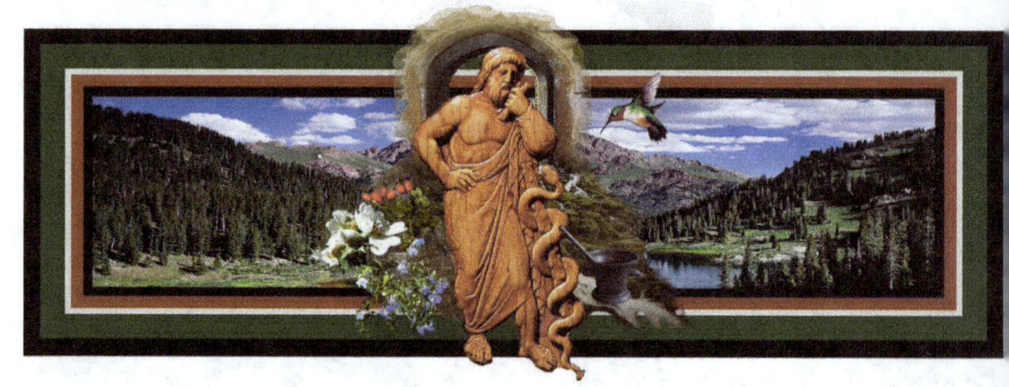

CURIOSITY
ITS ADVANTAGE & REWARD

In this work of healing bodies and bettering the world, there are certain qualities and propensities that tend to make us more effective at what we do — such as awareness, observation skills, and critical thinking,. But of these, most significant may be a quality for which all of humankind seems naturally endowed: *curiosity* – the exciting urge to uncover and discover!

It's something that starts when we're kids, and it's kids that often best embody this crucial characteristic, being as they are constantly curious, constantly drawn to the unrecognized and the unknown, enthusiastically exploring the new and the untested, delighted with exposing a world outside of the assumptions and conventions of parents and teachers. They tend to run in the direction of oddity and surprise, and unless something scares them they'll usually linger to examine each new thing, pondering every imaginable possibility.

The best healers – just like the best artists, the best scientists, and the best lovers – remain under the spell of qualities you've been endowed with since you were toddlers crawling on the ground, hanging upside down just to try out new perspectives, turning over every leaf to see what lies on the others side! Curiosity is a predilection that helps to increase understanding and aid us in personal decision making, by stimulating interest, increasing excitement and engagement, awakening passions, and triggering experimentation and creative application.

So what part does it play for herbalists, healers, and the co-creators of a better, healthier world?

Simple.   Without our relentless unflagging curiosity, we could slip into thinking that we already know all we need to about some plant or condition... thereby missing out on as yet unknown or even undiscovered actions and uses. Familiarity with a particular pattern is great, but it can also blind us to exceptions and anomalies, resulting in us failing to take into account the different ways that illness can present in different people.

Some long accepted "facts" can be just outright wrong, or at least not universally applicable, and yet there's a tendency to continue acting as if traditional maxims are reality until curiosity drives us to explore and challenge them.

We might accept biased interpretations of otherwise credible research, if we don't wonder what the hell might be mistaken, omitted, or slanted to make a particular case.

We will likely fail to notice how an herbal formula could be custom tweaked to account for the different constitutions of various people we try to help, whenever curiosity gets supplanted by protocol.

If we ever get bored and wish we were doing something else besides our herbalism, art or activism, it won't be because our work is any less significant, but because we have *ceased to be fascinated.*

There's no surer way to take the life and spirit out a healer's mission, than to "grow up" and lose one's curiosity to sober and often ill-informed adult "certainties."

Curiosity is the sparkling excitement and bright hope illuminating our work – the essential work of healing ourselves, each other, our communities, the society at large, and the precious natural world we are necessarily and irrevocably embedded within.

It's helpful to be aware of the many obstacles and challenges to curiosity, such as:

- A fear of the unknown, and of discoveries and realizations that could disrupt or discomfort
- Clinging to what we know, rather than risking being wrong and turning to what is yet to be revealed
- Fear of the responsibility to integrate and implement the things we realize or discover

Be aware of

- Attachments to a belief system and its dogma
- Making themistake of assuming instead of wondering
- Hyper-focusing to the exclusion of peripheral patterns and unplanned effects

Watch out for

- Your thought processes rigidifying over time
- Your ever taking new discoveries for granted
- Getting burned out – suffering that numbing of interest brought about by shit like exhaustion, or spending too much time at rote tasks and too little time with the plants

The way to treat or overcome such obstacles is a veritable voyage of exploration that takes us beyond accepted maps and templates into the netherworlds of fresh discovery and realization – made possible through the opportune tripping, fueling and enhancing of our curious natures.

The medicine we need to be better medicine makers, is the reopening of our minds and hearts to the unforeseen, the unexpected, the warp and weft of interconnection where each newly identified thread is a pulsing tendril leading to other entwinings, interrelationships, awakenings and revelations.

Just as there are obstacles and challenges to our native curiosity, there are also some definite aids & encouragements I can recommend.

First

- Recognizing the value of what is yet to be revealed, and the personal pleasure of discovery
- Intentionally seeking out and delving into the unknown and the unfamiliar
- Being open to the unfamiliar lying within that which you think you're familiar with
- Opening up to your emotional as well as intellectual assessments and responses
- Replacing "belief" with adaptable and evolving understandings

You'd be wise to

- Have some fun exposing, illuminating, or redefining the assumptions and beliefs of entrenched systems
- Embrace the discomfort of having *your own* treasured beliefs and assumptions augmented or flat out overturned
- And frankly, wise to reject *all* rigid dogma

I recommend you

- Give free rein to your many interests, exploring whatever attracts you
- Watch for the unexpected, rather than assuming the expected
- Explore that which others dismiss as unappealing or uninteresting
- Recognize when you engage things out of custom or social pressure instead of personal interest
- Follow a chain of interests from one to another, while trying to understand their relationships
- Take the time necessary to be explorative, spontaneous, and entertained

And especially

- Find creative ways to utilize and enjoy all that your searchings and discoveries reveal!

If your life, your herbal practice, your methods, activities or surroundings ever start to feel rote, predictable, boring, or "old hat," then I suggest that you get yourself a new hat, or else modify or repurpose what you have.

Like those children that I mentioned earlier, twist around or hang upside down until you can see things from a new angle, seemingly taking new shapes, juxtaposed against a different color and landscape. Allow yourself to delight in alteration, experimentation, customization, and personalization.

Indeed, let there be *no herbal leaf unturned*: our eyes and minds opened to the possibility of not only different colors and tones, to realizations about actions or uses, but to whatever unimagined visage or knowing might be exposed, to the chance even that a flower faery might nest hidden beneath its leaves, or that a magical botanical scent might be released with that fateful turning, and in the span of some tiny creature's heartbeat, redirect us to the enchantments of discovery and delight in the as-yet-not-known.

It's helpful for us to always approach things as if we were still beginners, no matter how many books we have either read or written, how many clients we may have helped, or how often something we think has been judged to be correct in the past. Look to each person or situation or place you seek to help, as if there are things still to be learned about them, pay attention to deviations, be prepared for surprises, allow yourself to be as thrilled by even seemingly minuscule, mundane or inconsequential discoveries as you were when first excited by the stories of bodily healing, by the curious smells of roots and flowers, by the clear summoning by imploring nature and its medicinal herbs.Our recovery, our redemption, our pleasure and satisfaction are all served by the same enlivened and unleashed curiosity that also propels the development of greater understanding and effectuality. We constantly improve, and constantly entertained and enriched, whenever we unleash our latent curiosities and follow them around the bend, through the concealing forest, on every scarcely marked track, certain there is always more for us to uncover, to plumb, to hear, to understand, to realize, and to actualize!

Join me, eager and agog, attentive and playful, keen as can be, gladly thirsting, aroused and hungering, as fascinated as a Seer or a child with the uncovering of everything's natures and nuances, by the endless shades and shifting colors and morphing forms, and by causes and consequences again.

Let us be drawn outside of our existing knowledge base by an un-categorizable music and the flapping of unseen wings just beyond what is visible — as possessed as we can possibly be by the enchantments of discovery and possibility once more.

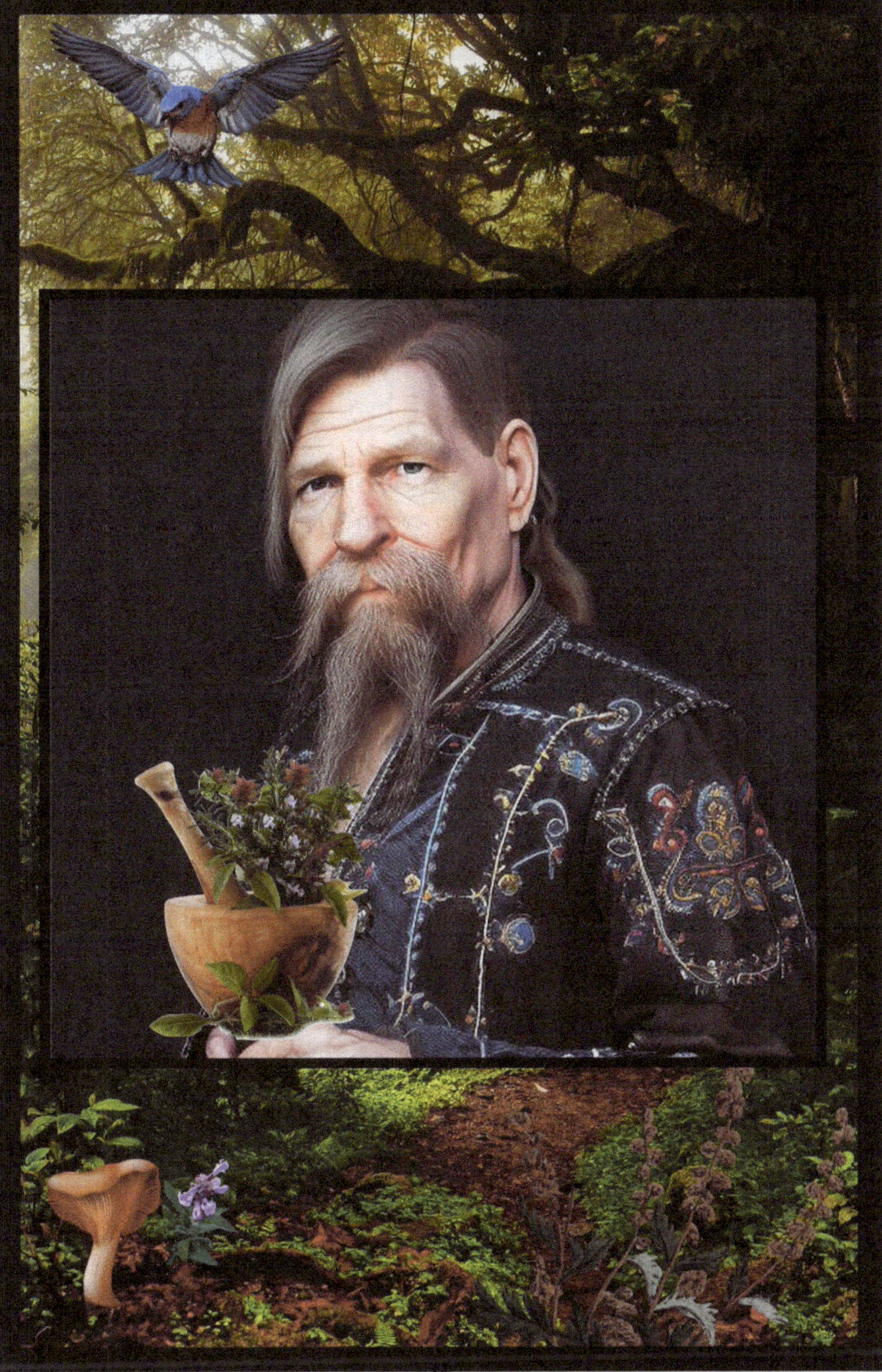

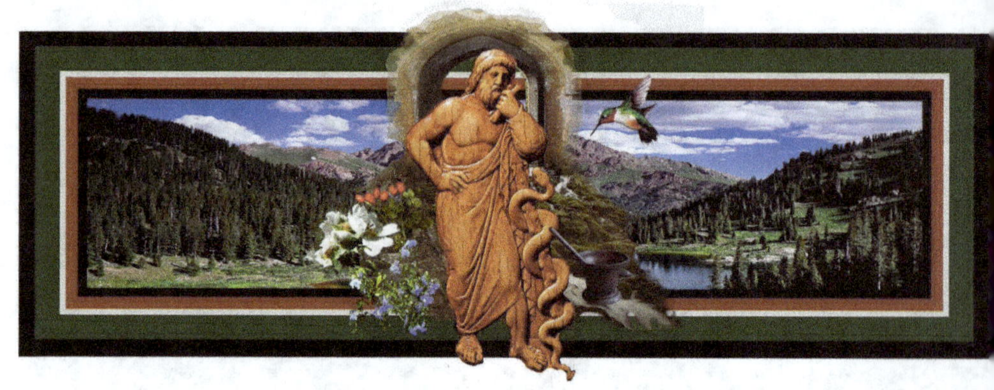

Heeding Your Calling
Accepting & Manifesting
Your Personal Healing Path

Tell me — do you sense something gnawing at your insides in what feels like an urgent plea for your attention? Do you sense a mission or purpose beyond and in excess of the work you once did and the life you once lived? Are there dreams or daytime visions that show up again and again like beckoning storylines whose plot arc you do not yet know, stories which you are somehow meant to help write? Do you see signs that seem to mark a lesser traveled path, signs that like guiding lights illuminate the most meaningful and amazing path ahead? When you quiet your mind and turn towards the unknown, do you seem to hear the rustlings of leaves, hear hints of otherworldly songs on the breeze, hear hushed voices that you can barely make out seeming to rise from the earth itself? Seriously, do you feel *called?*

The juncture of natural healing and plant medicine is labeled many different things. It's considered its own "field," although it overlaps with and utilizes elements of other fields such as botany, biochemistry, dietary studies, psychology, social justice, ecology and modern alchemy.   It's called a "science" by some people, since it utilizes scientific research and the scientific method of using sampling and controls to test hypothesis, and its called science even though natural healing has forever incorporated some of the essential precepts of ancient earth-centered spirituality.

It's referred to as a profession by some others, even though practitioners need not belong to any professional organization or meet any predetermined standards in order to practice their healing arts. It's said to be a "vocation" even when practitioners give their knowledge and herbs away as a service, spend their days helping the impoverished and marginalized, or are consumed with setting up free clinics at the sites of natural disasters.

What natural healing practices like herbalism are, if you haven't already guessed, is a *calling* — a call emanating not just from inside yourself but from the larger inspirited world of which you are an integral part. A calling is an urge that we can't shake off, an inner urge fueled by great external needs and unfilled roles. When we respond to its proddings, everything may seem to magically align in order to make our calling possible. And when we suppress or ignore it, we are likely to feel ill at ease, misdirected and unsatisfied.

A calling is a clarion, imploring you to step up and take on your most meaningful purpose. It's an assignment which you are particularly well suited to, a heart-touching imperative to which you must respond if you're to become all that you can be, the overwhelming imperative that you must act on if you're to make happen all that you are being gifted, impressed, equipped, instructed and empowered to do.

The doing is what it's all about. For example, you're not called to *be* an artist, a dancer or a healer, that's not what happens — you're called to *create*, to *dance*, and to *heal*. To be clear, callings are not about defining your identity and role, roles are something we're going to talk about elsewhere. A role is more like the personal form that your ways and means take, as you heed your calling and define your mission.

Every inborn talent and developed skill that you have, will be needed for the tasks and aims that you're being summoned to act upon. No matter how impossible your work or mission might seem, and no matter how exhausted you may ever feel, following your calling can mean that you're wholly actualized, that you're inspired and energized, thrilled and fulfilled, unbroken by any fears of challenge or inadequacy, that you're infused with an enlivening sense of direction, a feeling of excitement, expansiveness and light.

Your personal calling is not some general healer's conscription, but a particular, individualized, customized form meant specifically and ideally for you. It may mean utilizing a certain combination of approaches and practices, focusing on particular plants or conditions, serving a special group or need, or practicing in a certain community or physical place. No matter how it manifests in your case, your calling is something you have to volunteer for. It's not some magically inevitable fate, but a destiny that you opt for, a set of missions that you sign up for and are responsible for. It's something powerful that you're tasked with, that you naturally and happily assume.

If you are at all in doubt, ask yourself: Are you doing each day the most meaningful, healthful and impactful things that you can imagine? Or do your daily job and activities feel rote, bereft of excitement, insignificant or purposeless? Do you feel essential or peripheral, appropriately placed or *mis*placed? Well suited, or ill equipped? Inspired, or just informed? Stimulated, or only appeased? Wholly satisfied, or simply sustained? Directed, or aimless?

When we're truly heeding, we have no doubt that what we're doing in the moment is the very best thing possible, and we know in our very being that we are in the right place at the right time. We feel enriched even when we have little income. We feel recognized even if there are few persons who see us and our work for what we are. Neither social norms nor conventions can slow us down, as we move forward in our caring missions, dancing our way ever closer to the lilting songs of our imperative, towards the plaintive sounds of our Plant Healer's calling.

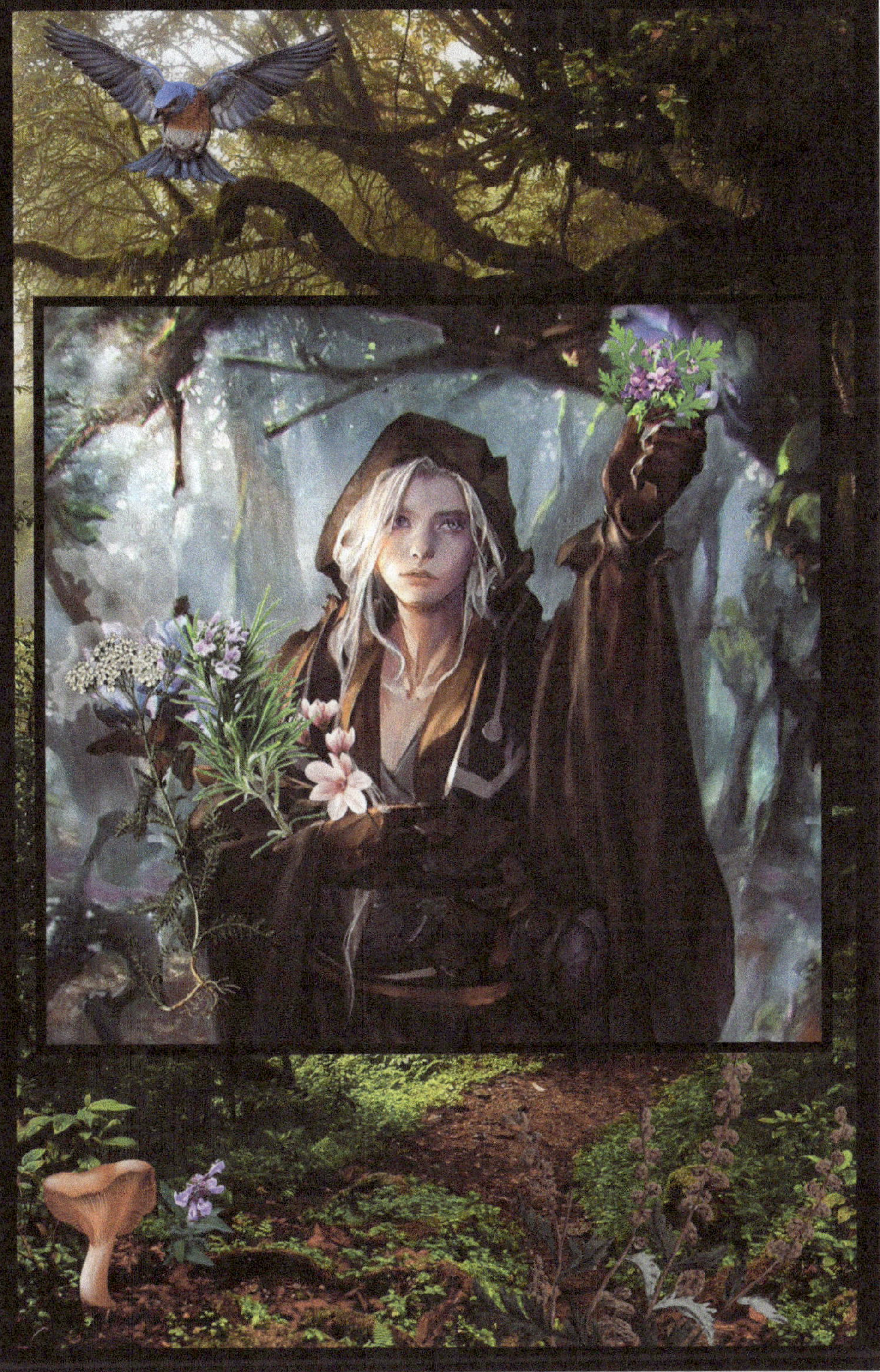

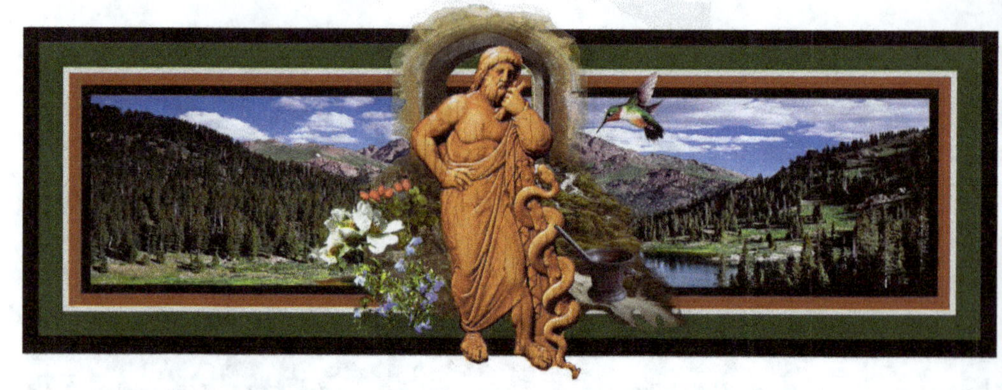

Finding Your Niche
What Best Distinguishes You?

Herbalists serve a general, collective medicinal role within the human community, assisting and contributing to people's health outside of the pharmaceutical and corporate paradigm. That said, every Plant Healer also has a particular individual medicine, a special repertoire of ways and means, a signature blend of qualifications that make each of us uniquely suited to a certain role, and that can ultimately determine what is our personal niche.

If I ask you now, you'd probably say that healing and plants are a big part of your purpose in life, but a healing mission is only manifest and actionable when we give it form. It needs definitive characterization, its own story, a target demographic to serve, a refined focus, and a particular set of harmonic approaches and methodologies, as well as dedicated means, platforms and venues.

Our purpose requires we choose and take on the responsibilities of a *role* within the larger healing intention and field. Which kinds of roles we take on should be determined by our interests and passions, and by our abilities, propensities, talents, and experiences — distinctive roles such as a folk herbalist, family herbalist or professional clinician. As a cultivator or forager, a producer of herbal medicines, a teacher, an artist, or a co-creator of a new healing culture.

Once we've determined our optimum role within our healing purpose, the next step is to sense and create our exclusive niche. The word niche comes from the Latin *nidus*, meaning nest, and as such it's a custom built, highly emblematic home place, the illustrative place that defines us and from which we act to help the world. We create a nest unique to each of us, a next by which we become known. It's woven out of the branchings and elements of the whole of our healing purpose and roles — a niche that we imagine and then construct specially for ourselves.

A niche is a subset of your chosen role, a type of specialization indicating not only your focus but your sensibility, aesthetics, personality, techniques and means. There are, for example, limitless diverse forms of folk healing, but your niche within that would be distinguished by a signature blend of influences, understandings, languages, and practices. As producer of plant medicines, your niche might be defined by your concentration on topicals or tinctures, on particular groups of herbs, on formulas all aimed at a certain class of diseases or conditions, on particular traditional or innovative ways of preparing the medicines, and on a certain branding feel that graphically evokes who you are and what you are all about. The role of herbal clinician can be claimed by many, but you will be known and sought out for the personal ways in which you practice, the convictions or beliefs you hold, your demeanor, the kinds of clients you choose to serve, if you concentrate on women or children, and the vibe you put out in your branding and promotion. A grower may limit their farms or gardens to herbs with the highest demand, to endangered species of plants, to exotic or local varieties, and they're further recognized for the exact ways that they cultivate, for the land that sculpts as well as empowers them, and for the story that they tell about why and how they do what we do. Teaching plant medicine is a widely valued position, but nobody is just a general teacher, generic or standard — we carve out a niche in this coveted role by becoming especially informed and adept in specific subjects and skills, by the ways we present and teach, and through the persona we project.

Specializing is how we are distinguished from and keep from stepping on the toes of all the other herbalists or plant people. To be successful or effective, a niche has to appeal to a particular audience, clientele, or market. It's determined as much by the kinds of people drawn to it, as it is by what you put out there. It's hard for the public to distinguish one generalist from another, or to parse different business names that all begin with the word "herbal."

The most viable and promising herbal practices will be those that address specific kinds of people and needs, in specific recognizable ways, with a memorable name and logo, a unique or unusual angle, a characteristic intention, look, tone and flavor.

The word niche is sometimes conflated with "nook" or "cranny," but it is both linguistically and practically closer related to an opportune positioning, the nest as aperture, a home-place vantage point with a clear view of and access to the world that we want to impact and assist. If we do well in our various Plant Healer roles, it will not simply be due to our capacities, efforts or good fortune, but because we've found — and then assertively staked-out — an inimitable and noteworthy niche that makes it all possible.

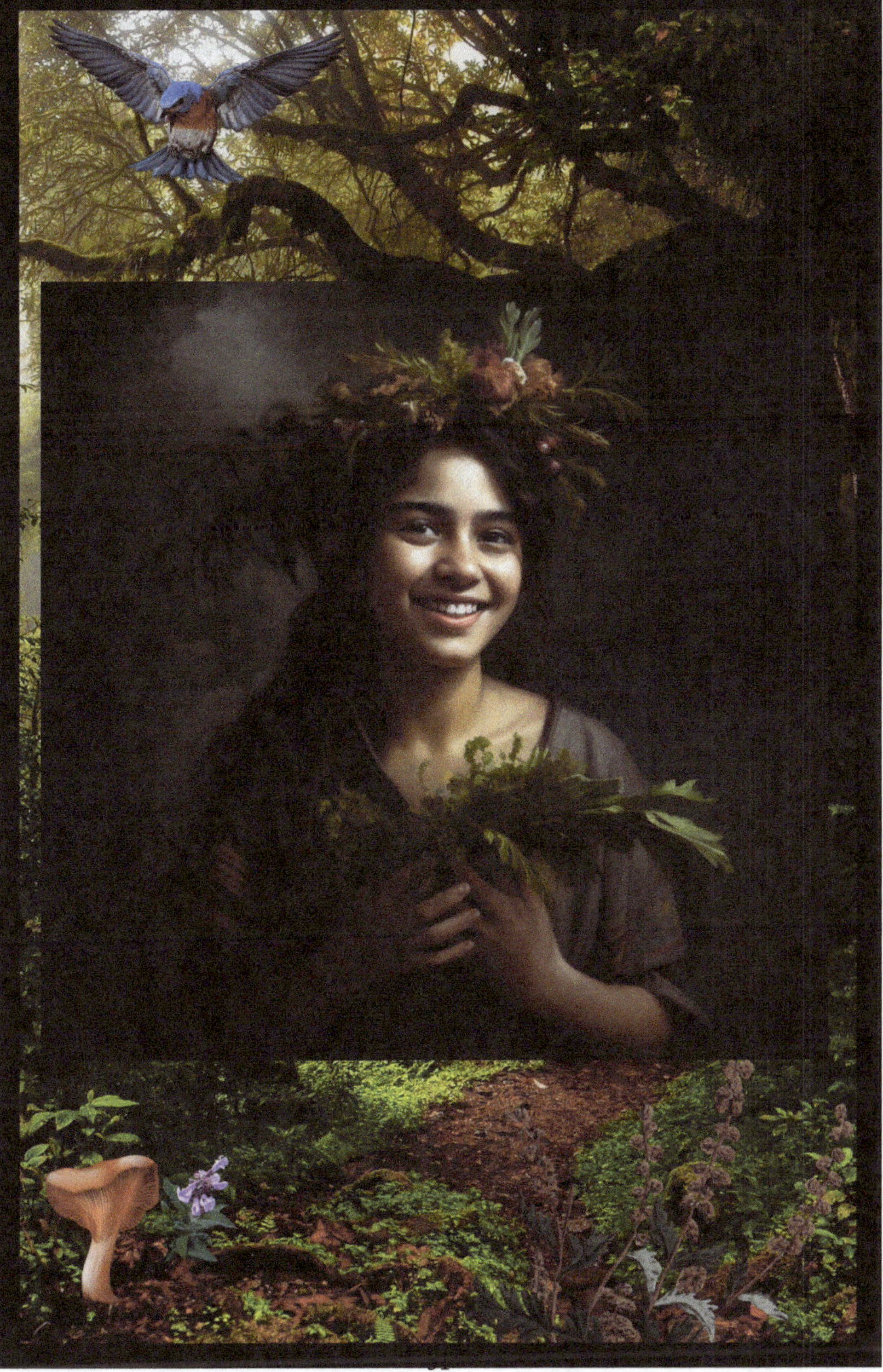

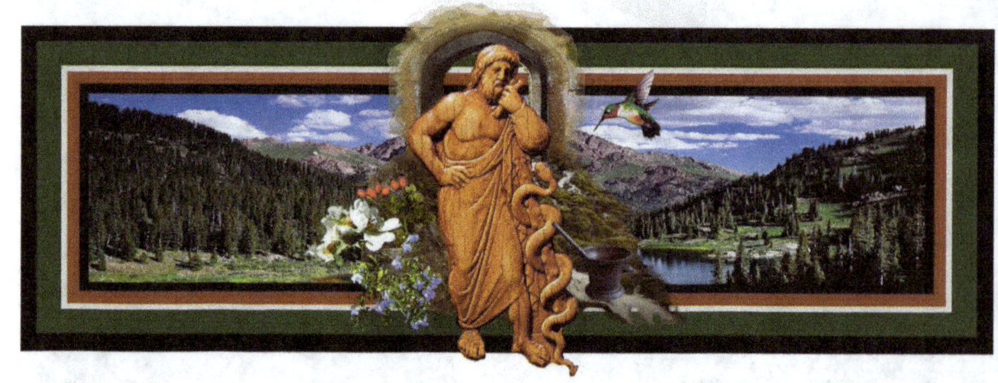

There Ain't No
Master Herbalists

Let's be clear right from the start: there's simply no such thing as a "Master Herbalist" — and there ain't no point in bullshittin' ourselves about it.

Yeah I know… it can be reassuring on some level to imagine that there are humble enlightened masters determining the course of herbalism and world events from beneath a magician's cowl or wise woman's cloak, moving often unseen through the busied throngs, or casting their well intended spells from behind a leafen screen of branches and brambles. When we consider the obvious limits of our own earned knowledge, it can be comforting indeed, comforting to believe that there exist individuals who've somehow managed to reach the very heights of wisdom and ability. But alas, it was totally certified and papered medical doctors who misdiagnosed and almost killed me, and a naturopath and a kitchen witch who resolved or alleviated most of my health issues.

If we think that it's possible for us to become masters of something, we're more likely to spend huge amounts of time and money seeking "official" recognition of it — even though there is no special anointed council, no friggin' cabal of superior, ascended, all knowing beings who can credibly make such a divine proclamation, and this is true no matter how much money we might pay, or how well we might do on their qualifying tests. There's no royal court where we can get knighted, no gilded venue where we're granted special favors and dispensations, so there's damn little reason for us to bow our heads, to hold our tongues, or to take a bended knee!

And if we think that we're *already* masters of something, it becomes sadly much easier to imagine that we've already secured all the information and skills that are needed for this important work of helping and healing. By thinking we're masters, we're stripped of much of the impetus to experiment, of the urge to explore and to adapt, stripped of much of our natural drive to continue with the vital formative processes of learning, developing, and evolving.

A Plant Healer is among other things, a lifelong student of all that our mentors, our personal experiences and *the herbs themselves* can teach us. There's no end to the countless lessons that we're afforded, no conclusion to or graduation from life's ever unfolding curricula, no ultimate plateau whereupon we can smugly retire or rest on our credits and laurels — not if we're on a constant chosen path of improvement, effectiveness, and fulfillment. The most knowledgeable, creative, effectual, beneficent practitioners I've ever met, have almost all been quick to point out what they *don't* know —- and have demonstrated an excitable eagerness to find out new things, to discover new patterns and possibilities, and to try new approaches... every single day that they're on the planet. They look at their many accumulating pieces of knowledge as contextual elements, not as immutable dogma. Every verifiable "fact" is viewed like building blocks, as filaments connecting to the limitless processes of a wondrous, never static, never fully understood universe.

It is entirely possible — and in many way it's necessary — for us to learn the foundational basics from which our practice can grow. But foundations are literally and metaphorically *concrete*, solid, strongly formed and largely unchanging. They are the opposite of a plateau of any kind, they're the actual base upon which we build, the principles we secure ourselves and our work to. They're what our characters, work and missions are built upon, but it is our continuing education, constant improvement, self realization and accomplishment that marks us.

The word "foundation" derives from the Old French "fundare," meaning to "lay a base for." It is thus the underpinning, the bedrock, the groundwork, the basis from which our full realization as healers *starts, not ends*. A foundation is defined as being "load bearing," and for the Plant Healer that load is the weight of all that we do and become. It's the very soil beneath us, the mycorrhizal-laced substratum from which we grow, act, stretch, and reach.

The word "master" is of course sometimes applied to someone with advanced abilities at some art or profession, but the dictionary also defines it as "having authority and control," as in the regrettable term "master and slave." It's also defined as someone having "complete knowledge," which I'm here to tell you, nobody ever does!

You don't need to be given authority in order to be a good herbalist. It's a mistake to think your bundle of knowing is ever complete. And you have no control the practice of healing, just the opportunity to help heal through your ever expanding awareness and ever deepening experience, through endless new insights and their caring application.

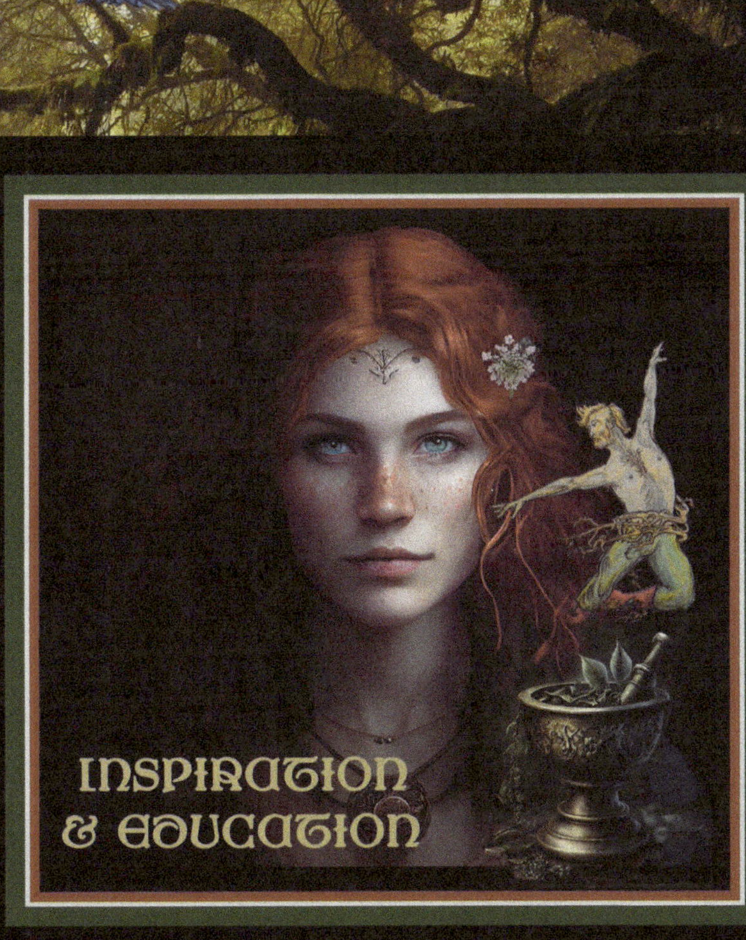
INSPIRATION
& EDUCATION

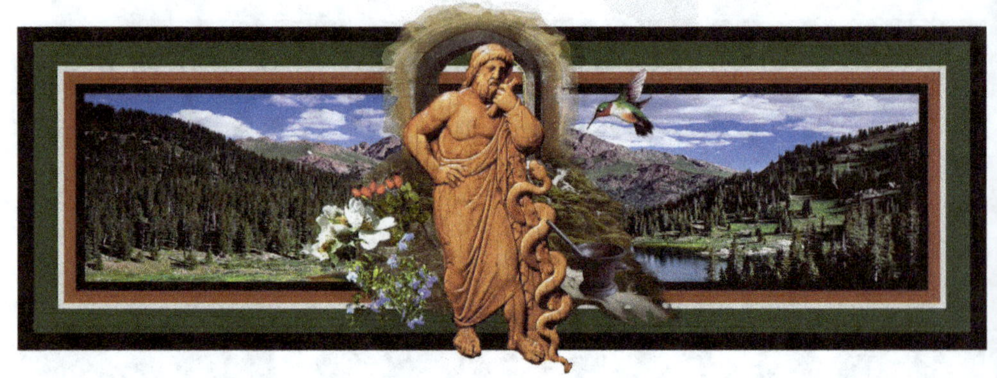

10 Traits
of a Great Herbalist
The Psychlogy of an Effective Healer

While there's really no such thing as a "master herbalist," there is certainly an increasing number of highly effective, highly adaptable herbalists that I don't at all mind calling great. And becoming greater – larger, better equipped, more insightful, more efficacious — is an entirely realistic and attainable goal for any of you committed to doing the healer's work. It's *great* to advance our knowledge and increase our abilities, to attain a foundational understanding from which we can further develop, and to be able to serve as mentors and inspiriteurs as well as caregivers.

I've previously described 10 areas of study that help make it possible to improve as healers. Now we're going to talk about 10 personal traits that we can work on developing and strengthening in order to become ever greater at the healing missions that each of us has chosen.

1. Awareness, Noticing, Interest & Curiosity

We all are born with degrees of awareness — awareness of our bodies and our needs, of our native strengths and weaknesses, our fears and dreams. And we all start with a natural capacity for awareness of our environs, from potential dangers to available pleasures. The part that we can grow and develop is the actual conscious noticing — discerning a thing or a need, a plant or an action, a relationship, a cause or a consequence, and distinguishing it from the vast field of elements it's bedded in.

56

Important is not just the number of relevant things you notice, but the *depth* of your awareness of them. The more you get to know them, the more lessons and blessings you're given, and the more able you are to utilize them in your understandings and your practice. Similarly, we start off as kids with a curiosity about everything. Every discovery, no matter how small, is generally followed up immediately by inquiry — a bubbling up of seemingly endless exploratory questions. The most minute or commonplace of things still manage to appear interesting, each and every thing housing some aspect or message or purpose yet to be revealed. To the degree that we lose that in adulthood, we lose the impetus to explore and the drive for discovery. The curious student of life is forever learning new things, and the practitioner who follows their interests is an effective and fulfilled practitioner indeed.

2. Enthusiasm & Passion

Following our interests is what leads most of us into any field or endeavor, with an interest in plants and an interest in helping people being a primary motivation for most herbalists. But we also need enthusiasm for our studies, our work and our mission, if we hope to sustain or expand it. When that enthusiasm is coupled with a persistent hungering to know and to do, it's what we call a passion. And don't be fooled into thinking you need to appear strictly clinical, unemotional or contained in order to be a credible health provider. The more passionate we are about related interests and aims, the greater our education, efforts and results will be as practicing Plant Healers.

3. Sensory Engagement

When doing our best, we recognize and evaluate the world through the lens of our physical, primal senses even before we parse and evaluate stuff using our reason, logic, and other mental processes. We can identify plants and guess their actions often, by smelling them and placing them on our tongue. We can "sense" something is wrong even without thinking about it, since smells and tastes can provide advance warning about a lot of things that could harm us. And smells and tastes can provide pleasurable hints about what we should be trying, consuming, or giving out to family or clients.

Even when they don't immediately result in some discovery or realization, it is our ancient senses that reward us with many of the feelings and flavors that make our lives rewarding and our work enjoyable — like the tickle of a pine branch as we step deeper into a forest, the sweetness of a mint stem, or moving through a world awash in botanical bouquets.

4. Pattern Thinking

Living only in our heads can lead to disembodiment and disconnection, and yet, thinking in various ways are perhaps the next most beneficial Plant Healer traits. Many thoughts are observations narrated by — *given words by* — the mind, occasionally something as simple as a statement of recognition, identification or judgment. Such thoughts often remain a minimally useful script until the point where we connect a thing or subject to a larger contextual matrix, connecting them to each other and to possible future outcomes through the use of visualizations, pertinent questions, salient comparisons, and informed speculations.

There is nothing that can't be better understood within a patterning of subjects and contexts, organs and agents, qualities and symptoms, relationships and interactions, causes and effects, known histories and projected futures. And in fact, nothing is ever truly disconnected, only disassociated, and all topics and stories, all paths and means, all herbs and illness, have an influence on each other to one degree or another. Like the filaments of subterranean mycorrhizal fungi, if you tug on any single strand the whole of dynamic life shifts and vibrates and reorients.

5. Thinking Outside The Box

It's pretty crucial that we think about things — such as minds and bodies, different approaches and methodologies, diverse plants and habitats, diets and diseases — as interconnected and interactive elements functioning within a larger process or container, components of an evolving organic whole. Equally important, is not letting our thought processes, conclusions or reactions be limited to any single set of assumptions, traditions or methods. We can't be great at healing without growing our proclivity to explore, experiment, alter and adapt. Failing to trust ourselves, strict adherence to traditions and protocols, and the fear of trying new things, are just three of the many reasons why our thinking can get boxed in and held back.

6. Critical Thinking

The third essential type of thinking is critical, no pun intended. You cannot fully or accurately assess a thing or an idea without a critical evaluation of its weaknesses or problems, of its evident merits and its possible benefits.

Critical thinking is not just about exposing potential faults, but about determining helpful abilities, blessings and advantages. Critical thinking is a trait that help us figure out which action or direction to take among what are always myriad complex options.

7. Envisioning & Foresight

Besides assessing things in the moment, utilizing our foresight can be a mighty helpful characteristic. What are the possible longterm effects of a certain way of thinking, of an activity or lifestyle, of an herb or a treatment? What consequences or results should we remain on the lookout for, and what optimum outcomes can we hope and try for?

Like foresight, envisioning is the imagining of possible futures. The difference is that foresight names what might happen to us or around us, while envisioning is us purposefully painting a picture of what we want to happen, and of what we can do to manifest it.

8. Decisiveness

After critical assessment, careful evaluation, vision and forethought, comes choice and decision. No matter what the external conditions and factors, it falls on us to pick what we understand to be the optimal path, route, means and methods serving our needs, our service to others, and our dreams and desires. Everything we choose and do is our personal responsibility, because it's we who select from all the options, whether we are aware that we're making choices or not.

The trait of decisiveness means that our choices are made consciously, and as promptly as they are needed. Avoiding the responsibility of decision making can result in our being at the mercy of our ambivalence, and result in the stalling-out of our progress and projects.

9. Determination

Determination is defined as a "firmness of purpose," doing what it takes to accomplish some goal no matter how many the challenges. Determination is the insistence that can come from a strong sense of purpose or mission. In the case of herbalism, for example, determination is what's needed to do the Plant Healer's work in the face of limited social acceptance, extensive studies, encroaching regulation, and often minimal income. When we assist someone's recovery from a formidable health condition, it often requires trying multiple strategies, adapting different formulas, astute observation over time, and our resolute determination to keep on trying until we're able to help make things better.

10. Wonderment

There's no way I could leave out this empowering characteristic, the childlike ability to be amazed by the wondrous, and to find the amazing in the so-called ordinary. Wonderment works to keep you engaged, motivated, looking ahead, and feeling rewarded. It not only fills us with awe for the plants that we work with, but awe for the actual natural processes of healing, and for the deliberate caring part we play in it.

These 10 are not a set of requirements for entering the healing trade, and they're not some set of qualifications you need to meet in order to be considered worthy. What these are, are improvable attributes, useful tools, and enjoyable and fulfilling benefits. You can look at them as a nesting of traits that we're all born with to one degree or another, characteristics and ways of being that even the wisest and most advanced practitioner can continue to develop, and grow, and broaden and deepen, and fine tune to our loving purposes…. putting them to ever better use on our personal Plant Healer paths.

I hope you'll find this useful in your ever more meaningful life and practice. *It's gonna be great*…. and so, my friends, will be *you!*

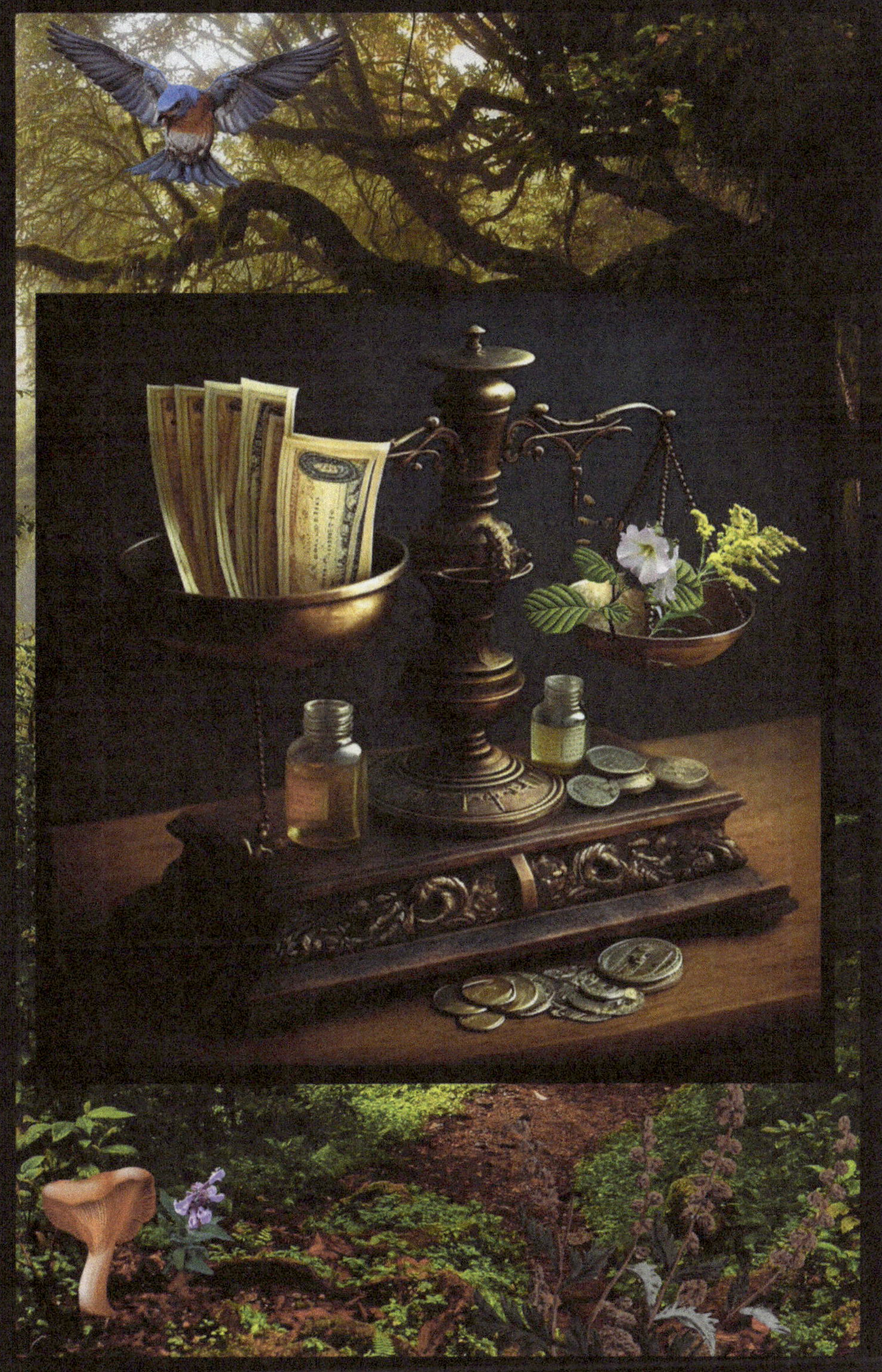

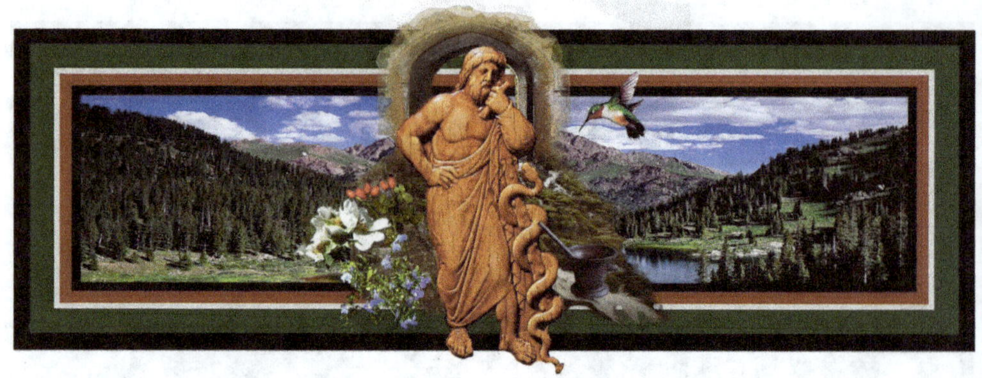

MONEY & HERBALISM
MAKING A LIVING,
& LIVING AS AN HERBALIST

We might as well get right to the point: If your main reason for getting into herbalism was to make big bucks, well — you pretty much messed up!

Some of the most satisfying and caring jobs, like being a conservationist or a grade-school teacher, get paid the *least*, and being an herbalist is no exception. Yet while you're not likely to ever get rich off of plants, you damn sure *can* earn enough income to meet your essential needs, to fund and enable your service to the community, and to make possible the richly living of your most meaningful dreams!

What is entirely possible, reasonable and *doable*, is to channel your obsession with plants and healing into an income-producing lifestyle, making your living from work that reflects what you are most interested in and best at. The various forms this can take can include:

- Seeing and advising paying clients
- Cultivating and selling medicinal plants and fungi
- Making and marketing your own formulated herbal preparations
- Starting an online herbal products business
- Opening a brick and mortar apothecary
- Writing and marketing herb books
- Teaching classes about herbs and healthcare
- Even launching your own online or physical herb school

All of these endeavors provide opportunities and ways to generate some money doing what we love. At the same time, we'll also be rewarded by the gratitude of everybody we help, and by our intimate working relationship with the healing green beings. We'll reap the benefits of time in the close company of plants and nature, the benefits of reawakened wonder and exciting new discoveries. We'll be given bonus pay in the currency of leaves' tastes and flowers' scents, in knowing what our purpose is, and in giving our all to our personal chosen mission.

In the case of Plant Healer publications and events, I can tell you it's far more of a mission than a well managed business. We've made it likely that we'll forever have to stretch to cover food and bills, by prioritizing providing immense amounts of articles in Plant Healer Quarterly magazine over sending out what could be smaller, more profitable editions; by releasing a free monthly Herbaria zine especially for financially challenged readers; by making the annual Good Medicine Confluence events about building community more than about putting money in our pockets, and by awarding a helluva lot of scholarships to those folks most in need of encouragement.

Our family may not be able to afford medical insurance, but our choice of career and sense of mission means we are forever happy with what we do. We're forever feeling rich belonging to such a supportive herbal community, living in such a wild place as our rewilded Anima Sanctuary, feeding our passions, and giving to the world in all the many ways that we can!

A big part of our Plant Healer work is showing you that you can be who you really are and most want to be, doing what matters most to you. We teach that "making a living" is only but a single practical aspect of what it means to make sure we are each, at all times, fully and wholly alive. For these reasons and more, I say "go for it!".

If your dreams are to be able to survive as a dedicated, full-time herbalist, hear me now — *your dreams can come true!*

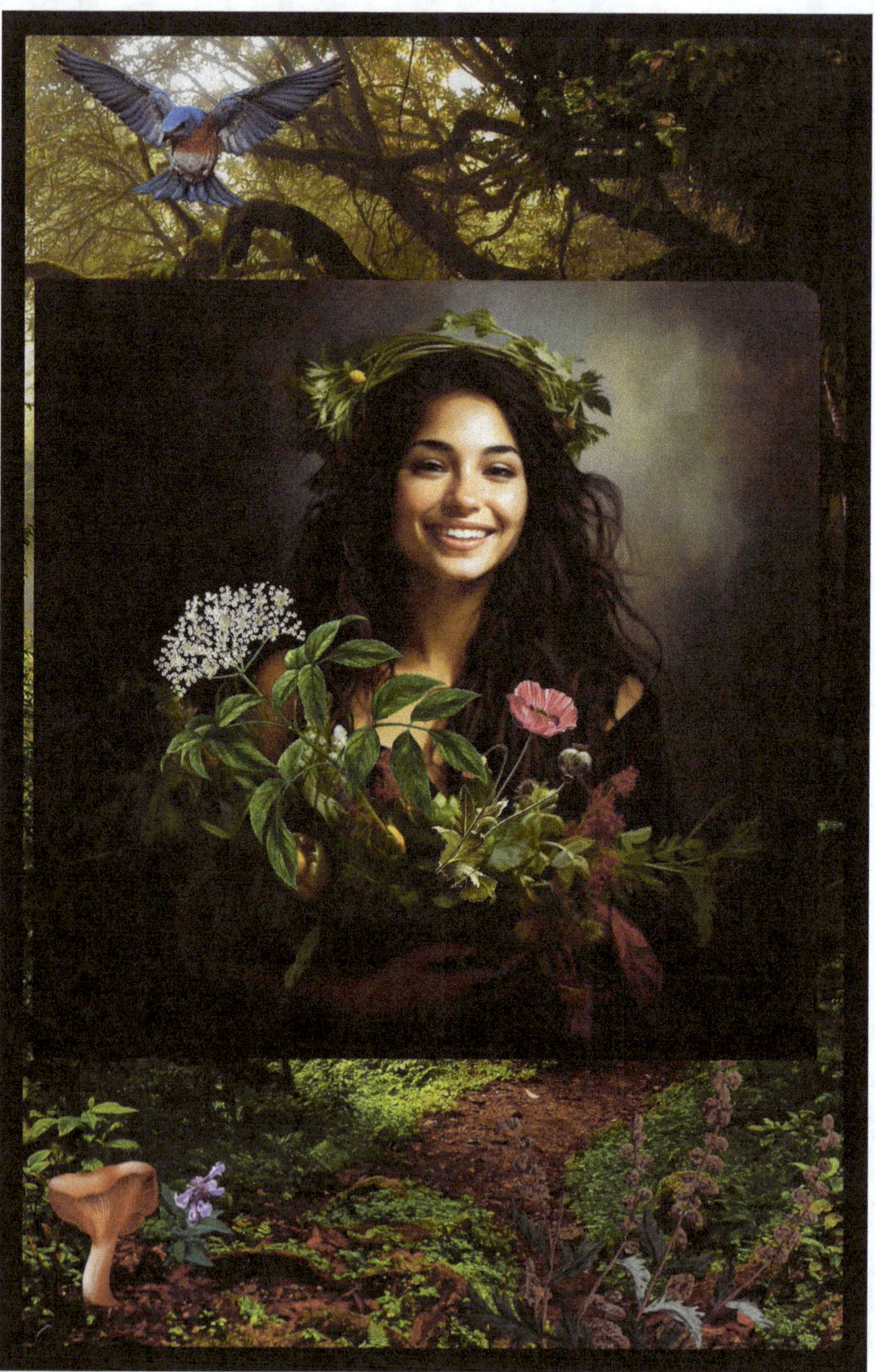

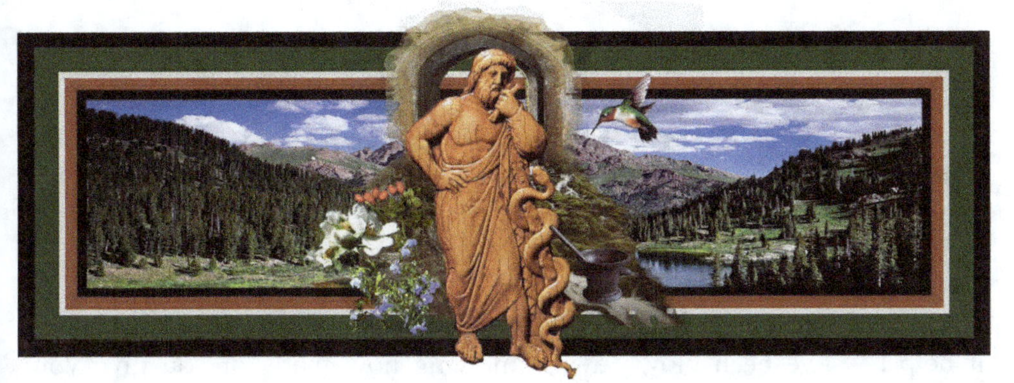

BEING OF SERVICE
GIVING BACK – FROM HERBALISTS'
SLIDING SCALES
TO VOLUNTEER WORK

Folk herbalists and other natural healers like yourself get into this work out of a strong sense of wanting to *be of service,* to do good for the world, often one person at a time. You want to help those who are in pain, and you want to use herbs and methods that spare them the side effects of prescribed drugs. You've made a pledge to live and practice in ways that honor the plants as well as the healing processes, and you intensely care about making things better. While you both deserve and need a substantial income in order to survive and do your good work, your heart's calling is likely centered around and anchored in a poignant sense of serving.

This is unlike most M.D.s these days, doctors whose desire to ease suffering is often compromised by their desire for the dollar and the push to get patients in and out the door as quickly as possible. While they might be genuinely happy to see people recover, their system is based on everyone being able to afford insurance, and so there's damn few who offer reduced rates or deferred payment plans to those most in need.

In my years of working with herbalists and hosting the Good Medicine Confluence, I've always found myself impressed with how many of them offer discounts to different individuals and demographics, or dedicate a portion of what they make to a community or cause. Again and again I've witnessed herb shop owners giving out lengthy free advice, heard the tales of Plant Healers staffing free herbal clinics at festivals and gatherings, and watched our Confluence teachers hand out tinctures to attendees saying "send the money when you can," or "just see if it works, and pay me later if it helps!" I've been blown away knowing how many of you give your "spare" time to repairing plant habitat, launching community gardens with healthy food crops and medicinal herbs, or offering consultations at a local free clinic. I work mighty hard to support and champion the Plant Healer tribe, but how could I not, when you all care so deeply and give so much?

Compassionate service is partly corrective and redemptive, but it's not just what redeems us a species, it's something that actually helps keep the great energetics wheel going round. It is literally "doing a good turn." The entire natural world is part of an interactive gifting cycle, constantly revolving, and in which all things give and receive in overall equal measure... but *service* is something more, in that it's an actual conscious choice, a deliberate and not at all automatic gifting. It means extra to the recipients that your service benefits, because it's recognized as being an intentional and heartfelt expenditure of your time and skill, your medicines and your love.

This is true whether you're a neighborhood practitioner or a large and growing company, a medicine maker or consulting clinician. The ways and means may be different, depending, but the motivation for service, the call to contribute to wellbeing or justice — and the powerful and admirable desire to give — is the same.

I'll give you here just a few of the possibilities, for inspiration.

Herb sellers, herbal clinicians, herbal consultants, and other kinds of natural healers can serve by offering things like:

• Sliding scales, offering from a small discount, down to totally free for those who could in no way afford to get help otherwise. This can be based on whatever criteria feels best to you, and be for whatever kinds of people or situations you feel strongest about.

- Deferred payment plans can be a way to help people out, while still getting some funds coming in instead of bearing all the costs of labor and supplies.

- Work trades can sometimes be a way for recipients to feel good about giving back to you. You provide treatments, medicines, consultations and followups, educational classes or whatever your specialties happen to be, and they in turn provide a service like helping with your medicine making or stocking shelves, or even childcare or vehicle repairs!

- Bartering is the oldest and most natural of human economies, and long before there was any currency there were folks trading their labors or surplus resources for someone else's skilled help or stash of curative herbs. Those without the money to pay you, will feel especially well served by an offer to accept barter.

- You can volunteer some of your time every month, often doing what you love — from offering to help at a free clinic on certain days, to projects like planting endangered plant species on public lands, and even non-herbal related labor for organizations and communities that you want to support the goals of.

- Donations of medicinal herbal products to aid groups and nonprofits is an awesome way to gift, especially during difficult times or following some natural disaster.

- And donating a percentage of profits to a group, a project or a cause, is a simple way to contribute, supporting the people, the issues, and land that you love.

If you happen to have a company of any kind, a school or apothecary or herbal product business, you might additionally consider the following ways of serving:

- Providing discount programs and products for those you want to assist and support, such as the marginalized or the indigenous, as well as for the impoverished.

• If you have a physical or online herbal school, or organize educational events, scholarships are a great service, encouraging and equipping folks who have the interest and passion but can't get the bucks to pay.

• You can dedicate a percentage of company profits to selected groups that are doing the most for what you value the most, helping to fund things like health education programs, social justice causes, organic farming initiatives, seed banks, food banks, land trusts, botanical sanctuaries, and conservation organizations like the United Plant Savers.

• You might think about giving your employees paid time off to participate in meaningful volunteer work, those they help will appreciate and they employees may love the opportunity to do something different as well as beneficial.

• And lastly, no matter what kind of business you have, you can well serve the community, spread herbal awareness by becoming a sponsor of one of the many annual herbal events like the Good Medicine Confluence or Breitenbush.

You know how a spiritual ceremony is sometimes called a service? In this sense, any of the above way we might give are a spiritual devotion, a selfless sacrament, a liturgy of empathizing, aiding and remedying. A Plant Healer's service is always more than pragmatic assistance. It can be seen as an act of kindness, as a warm helping hand, as encouragement and equipping, and as devoted ministration.

Increasingly, you know how to "be of service." You're a caregiver, for sure, but you don't just *care*, you're indisputably *givers*. It has never been more evident how very much you give to others, never more clear than how much you benefit this living, needing world.

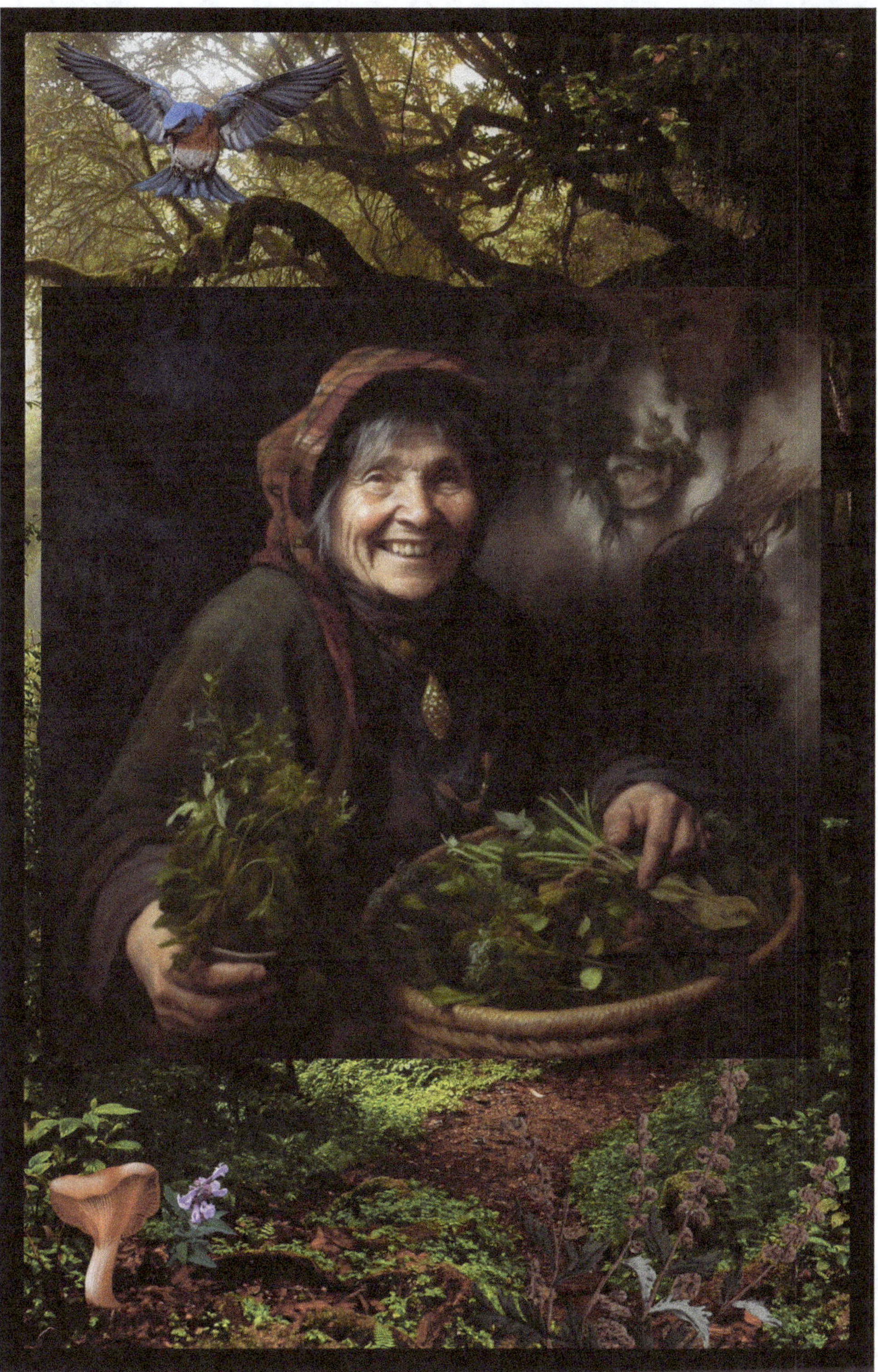

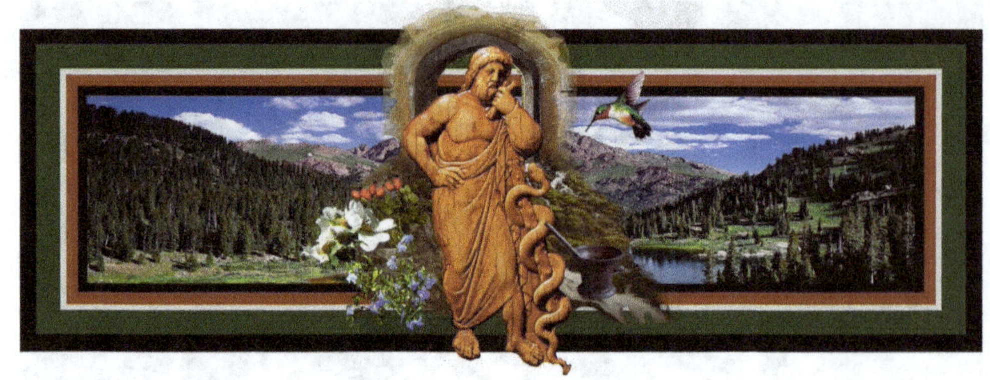

10 CHARACTERISTICS OF A CARING HEALER

I recorded a Plant Healer Path video about the "10 Traits of an Effective Herbalist," outlining the practical psychological elements that I consider most useful for a practitioner of virtually any sort. You'll note that none of the aspirational traits I listed there are ideological, and it's important to understand that all of them can be further developed and increasingly utilized by anyone willing to make the effort. But this isn't to say that both we ourselves — *and* our healing work — couldn't benefit from the addition of some core moral characteristics.

By "moral," I sure as hell don't mean some simplistic unchangeable notion of "right" and "wrong," things like rightness and wrongness are way too complex and situational to set into proverbial dogmatic stone. Nor is this about "do"s and "don't"s. By "morality," I'm certainly not referring to medical taboos or exposed cleavage, adhering to rules or social conventions, or trying to live up to anyone else's expectations for you. Nor am I going to try to codify what methods or medicines are "good" and "bad," I'm only going to talk with you about some perspectives, values, and personal qualities that could aid us in making distinctions, evaluations, and determinations on our chosen paths. What I am referring to is a composition of traits which in concert can make it more possible for us to discern for ourselves what is best for us... and best for those that we seek to help.

Without any hesitancy, I can suggest the deepening and cultivating of the following:

1. Purposeful Self Awareness

The development of usable virtues begins with our self awareness: our recognition of what things we do out of benevolence, and of what kinds of things we do well — as well as identifying what it is we do poorly, and recognizing the things we do out of reactivity, selfishness, defensiveness, or anger.

We can develop these instrumental virtues by working on our missteps and challenges, along with making use of the talents and blessings that we're born with — paying attention to the ways that we can become better people and better herbalists, while simultaneously seeing ourselves for who we are right now, giving credence to the nature and totality of our beings.

2. Authenticity & Integrity

Authenticity rises to the level of a moral principle in an age when objective truths seem unattainable or unvalued, within a culture of vaulted artificiality and personal misrepresentation. With institutional medicine and giant pharmaceutical companies making false claims for their often harmful drugs, a natural healing enterprise stands out as a genuine caring mission, its practitioners motivated more by deep caring than by the potential profits. Herbalists tend to be some of the most genuine of people, genuinely being themselves, genuinely compassionate, offering genuine herbal products along with genuinely helpful advice.

Closely related to authenticity is *integrity*. Integrity is generally conflated with honesty, but it's really more the quality of being whole and undivided, with minimal moral and behavioral contradictions. It's about a soundness and internal consistency. It's being scrupulous, meaning diligently working to avoid being either dishonorable or unintentionally harmful.

The Plant Healer strives daily to be both wholly real, and really and truly whole.

3. Honesty

Honesty is another closely related quality and characteristic. While modern medicine has certainly done a lot to ease suffering and save lives, it has also been dishonest as hell. Herbalists, on the other hand, have almost never been the charlatans and uncaring "snake oil" salesmen that corporate propagandists have screamed about whenever needing to ensure their hegemony. The worst thing that most herbal practitioners have ever been is naive or overly hopeful. Unlike big pharma causing the death and debility of millions of patients, the Plant Healer is honest about the usually benign effects of herbs, and honestly does their best for their communities and clients.

4. Empathy & Compassion

Empathy is to feel some of what others are experiencing. This can sometimes be more of a mental recognition and understanding of someone's struggles and pains, and other times an actual physical sensation such as feeling an electrifying jolt when witnessing someone falling onto the hard pavement. In both examples, empathy is a characteristic to develop and use, a quality that can increase our sensitivity to what our friends and clients are fearing, confronting, suffering, or hoping for.

Empathy by itself, however, needs compassion to be actionable. It's theoretically possible to sense what someone is suffering yet still not really give a shit. Compassion is the quality of actually caring about these beings, caring about what they feel, caring about their health and wholeness and realization.

5. Kindness

Kindness is how we express and manifest our empathy and compassion. Friendliness and niceness can sometimes be just a formality, a simple politeness — but kindness, on the other hand, is a heartfelt gifting of some kind or other. A kind word, with the conscious intention to make someone feel better. A kind act that we believe will help someone do better or enjoy more. Kindness is a prime Plant Healer motivation, with their every herbal formula an act of kindness, and folks trust that they will be treated kindly when they go to a Plant Healer for suggestions or relief.

6. Patience

Don't think of patience as just a practical waiting or slowing down. It has a moral element, in that our impatience can hurt others at the same time it can abbreviate our assessments and reduce the chances of a lasting positive outcome. Being patient when learning can result in greater understanding. Patience with unresponsive or unresolved health conditions, can lead to more detailed observations over time, result in our figuring out improved approaches and treatments. Patience with ourselves proves essential as well, so that we don't become disheartened by any perceived failure to be all the help to someone that we want to be.

A good way to grow our patience is to work at *pacing* — striving for a continuous fluid tempo that neither races nor stops. There is a rhythm to healing, moments of intercession and moments of pause and contemplation, as well as moments of exertion and movement, and we do our Plant Healer dance best when we move in what dancers and long distance runners often call "the zone."

7. Awareness of The Energetic & Spiritual

Of great benefit is the characteristic of conscious bodily and energetic interconnection, intentionally connecting on myriad levels and in myriad ways to the people we hope to help — and connecting sensorially and spiritually to the plants themselves. This is a continuous process of tuning our hearts and actions to the immense symphony of the sacred, of regeneration, of the natural world, and of healing and wholeness specifically. In these ways, the Plant Healer doesn't just treat illness, but contributes to every manner of healing people and planet, contributing beauty, contributing love.

8. Generosity

Meaningful contributions and substantial service can be exhausting. We sustain our healing efforts through periods of rest and self care, but what feeds an herbalist's work more than anything else is often an overwhelming generosity. The Plant Healer is driven not only by people's needs and a desire to help, but by a generous spirit that drives us to give — to give our precious time to patients and pledges, to cares and causes. To give the knowledge we learn to others who can benefit from it. Give out our counsel and support, and ever so generously give our hearts.

9. A Code of Honor

The penultimate characteristic of the Plant Healer is the proclivity to create for ourselves — and then *live* by — a self-authored ethos, a personally chosen code of honor that can include things like: an adherence to justice, not hurting or taking advantage of those who are weaker or more disadvantaged, providing discounted or free service to the most in need. Things like cultivating scarce or endangered medicinal plants, being careful not to over-harvest when wildcrafting herbs, or refusing to cut corners when creating the most effective possible medicines. Social customs and regulations can be really screwed up sometimes, and deserving of our deliberate disobedience…. but a code of honor that we personally spell out and promise too, is something to stick with and never betray or compromise.

10. Devotion

These all lead us to devotion, our tenth valuable moral characteristic. Devotion is loyalty to a worthy idea, purpose, course of action, person or place. It is a commitment and pledge *kept*.

The Plant Healer is known to be committed to the work and its possible benefits to the world. Faithful to your principles. Devout, in your making of your practice into a defining sensibility, into what becomes a lifelong service and ever evolving ritual.

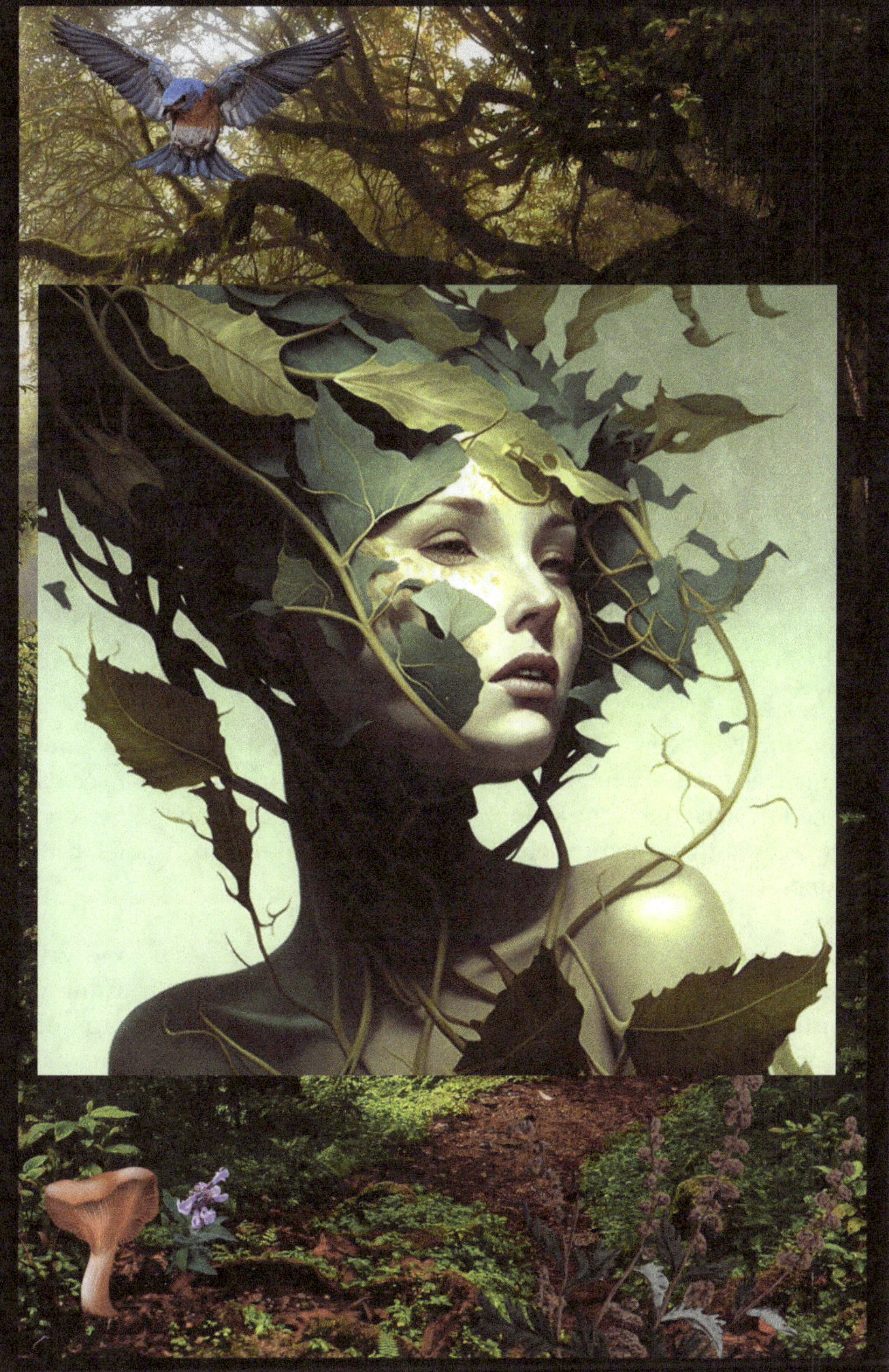

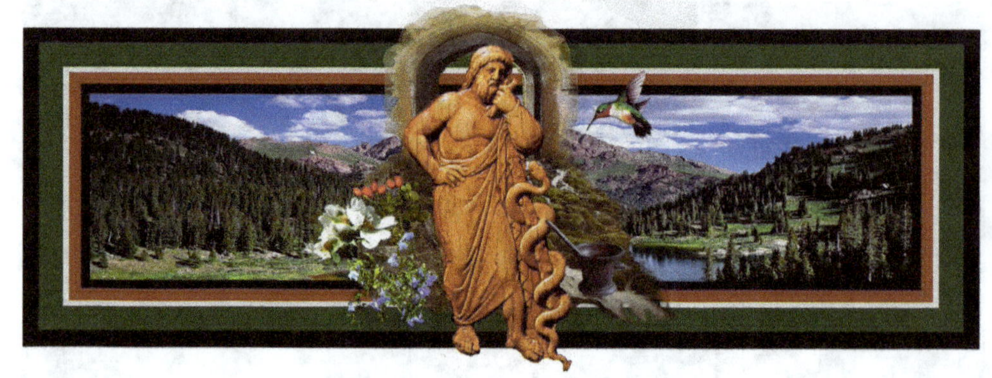

GLAD MISFITS
SOME BENEFITS OF
BEING UNBOXABLE

All my life I've been an advocate for the outsiders, the oddballs, and the marginalized, folks who through no fault of their own get rejected or sidelined by society. This can look differently depending on the person and whatever role they might seek to play, but let's take herbalists as just one example.

Healers who work with plant medicines were highly respected and valued for thousands of years, but then were increasingly dismissed starting with the institutionalization of health care and the hegemony of pharmaceuticals. Even now with herbal preparations getting hugely popular again, herbalists are still considered by many in society to be charlatans and freaks, seen as either old fashioned throwbacks or alt-culture weirdos.   Herbal accreditation and professional organizations are in part a reaction to herbal practitioners being treated like fluff-cakes or outsiders by the medical establishment, but even even herbal organizations themselves can inadvertently add to the ostracization to the degree that they discredit uncertified "folk" healers as if they're anything less.

I personally don't feel sorry for the marginalized, so much as care about and admire them. I see in them stories often far more interesting than the commonly accepted narratives. There's much to be appreciated about the very qualities and characteristics that make it so extra difficult for them to fit in, but this doesn't mean that they actually enjoy feeling excluded, or that they chose their place on the far outskirts. The marginalized are shoved to the edges for a number of reasons, but it's seldom because they actually want to be. Similar to what the system does with products on a conveyor belt, anyone who deviates from the standard or template can be considered flawed and tossed aside before societal packaging.

Misfits, on the other hand, often make a conscious choice to reside on the margins, seeing it more as a magical hedge, as the boundaries and entranceways to an Otherworld of possibility and reimagining. Misfits are the marginalized, but with the addition of agency and attitude! We tend to feel good about growing ourselves without bending to external rules and templates. We often take pride in being labeled as "different," and get a kick of "breaking the mold." It might feel like our calling or dream to sculpt an identity and life that sets us apart. Or it may simply feel like it's worth it to be true ourselves no matter how uncomfortable it makes us, what challenges it presents, the penalties or the cost.

There's obviously a price to be paid for being an outlier, whether we're a deliberate maverick or not. If we're not a typically functioning part of some machine, there's many of its benefits we're not going to have. There are no "help wanted" listings for unique job descriptions and previously unheard of approaches, and there are fewer options for earning a steady income for anyone bringing unusual interests and talents to the table. Supposedly individualistic art and music are a lot harder to market to people if they don't easily fall into a known genre or existing trend. We may be penalized for being neither a typical "professional" nor a factory worker, denied funding because of our beliefs, get fired from a needed day job because of how we dress or wear our hair. We might be shamed for not belonging heart and soul to a single major religion, or for not being totally in one political camp or another, we can could be either preyed on or ignored. There's no gettin' around it, it can sometimes feel lonely at the edges.

But oh, the benefits!

Benefits like: Honoring yourself by honoring your deepest needs, honoring your particular or even *peculiar* gifts, and honoring your visions. Benefits like no longer having to repress or submerge your most real identity, your personality, your beliefs or aims or missions. Like getting to choose doing what feels right to you, rather than just doing what some authoritative entity requires of you. Like not having to compromise your ethics or your tastes to fit in. Like never having to feel like "a round peg in a square hole," and never again having to deny some essential part of yourself just to be accepted or approved.

There is an old saying that describes anyone going their own way: "marching to a different drummer." I prefer to say someone "dances to a different drummer," since marching usually requires taking orders and getting in step — whereas even a choreographed dance is at its core a fluid and very personalized expression of who we are, how we feel, and what we care about. Being considered strange is like the opening steps of our individual, signature dances, a dance of the exceptional and extraordinary, of the distinctive and remarkable, the unpredictable and uncanny, the memorable and unmistakable.

Think about it. Natural health practices that have been dissed as unconventional have proven to be some of the most effective. The most effective medicines are often formulas and protocols that are uniquely tailored to each client. Being considered weird can be more a matter of being puzzling and bedazzling. Incongruous can be a chance for the unexpected. Peculiar is not only uncommon but irregular, custom, personal. As soon as we figure this out, being considered an oddball or misfit starts to sound like a compliment.

This is not to say, however, that we can't ever hope to *belong* — belong to some shared union, to a clan centered around a set of values, an alliance of purpose, a sharing of knowledge and skills, a dedication to a sound, a style, or a beautiful, wished-for result. The healthy way to fit into anything is like a kid's puzzle, with each and every piece unique and different from all the rest, and yet with there being a way in which their particular exacting curves, inimitable recesses and protrusions can virtually key into those surrounding it.

We easily may feel outside of things, marginalized, even isolated. And yeah, we may feel lonely from time to time — but *we are never alone.* We are united as Plant Healers by our love for nature, for plants and their lessons. We're naturally brought together by our overwhelming desire to help ease suffering and make the world a better place. And beyond that obvious alliance of aims, we're also integral elements of something truly unusual and valuable, each of us with our own home bases and ways of serving, contributing our own thoughts and visions, forms and angles, rhythms and tones. You and I are part of a league of misfits, of wondrously unboxable medicine beings and medicine makers, We're the delighted deviants, vital participants in a caring and creative coalition of culture shifters, the devoted lifelong members of what is truly a marvelous misfit tribe.

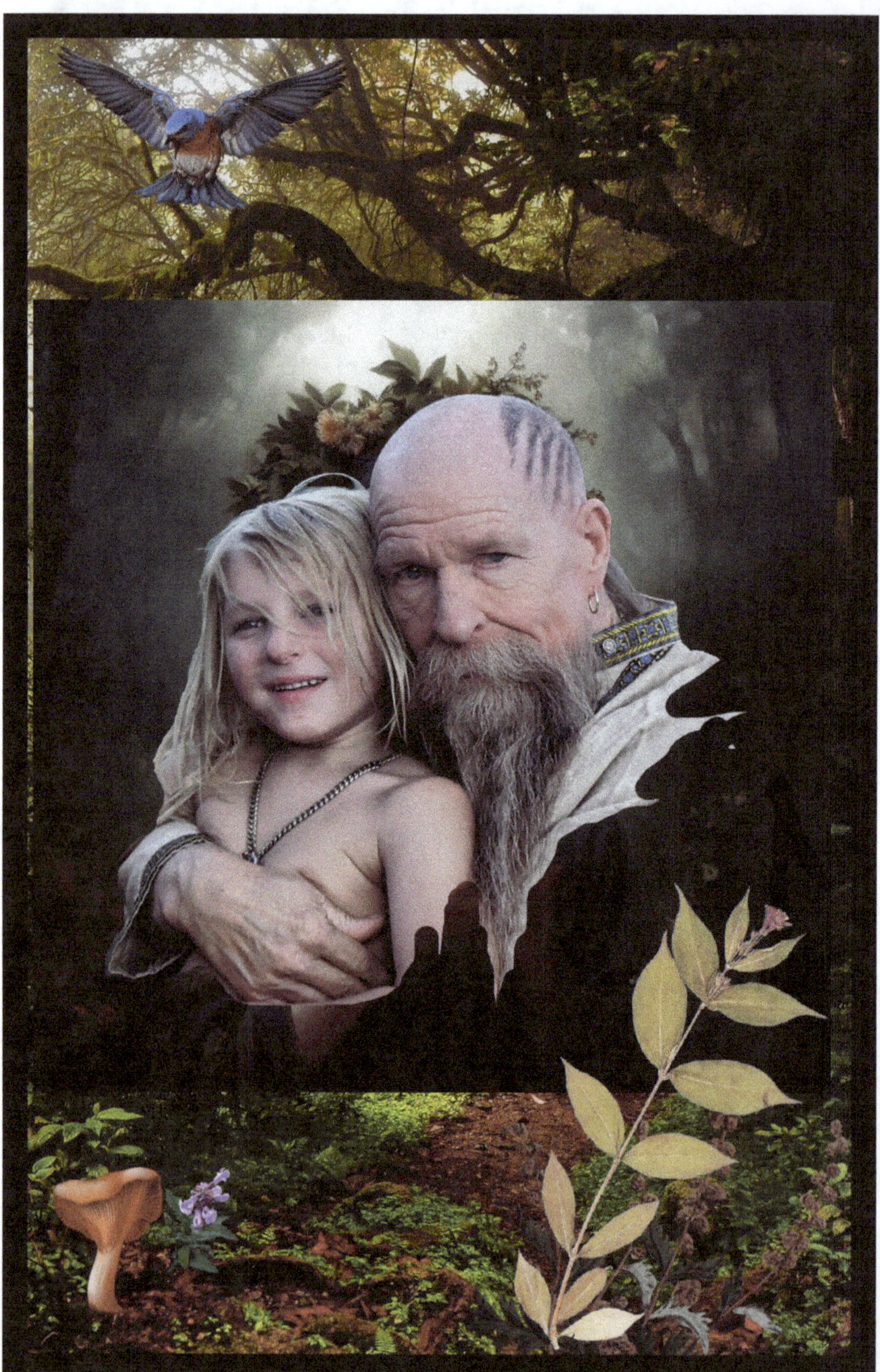

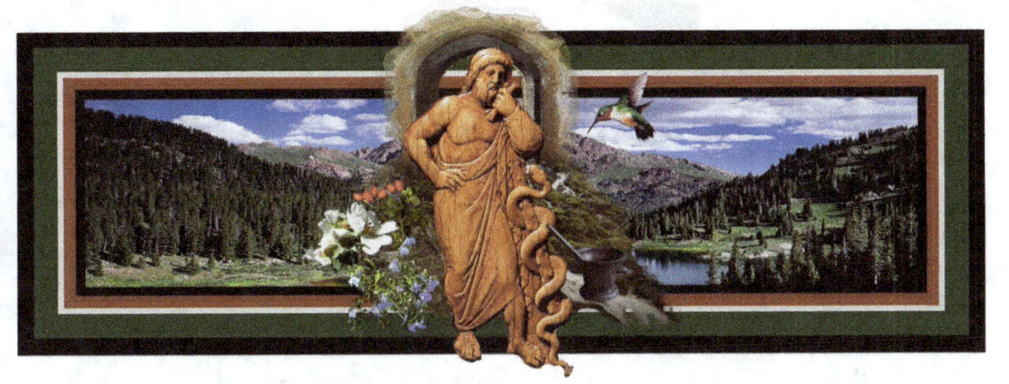

Herbal Family
Relationships & Alliance

When we read about the realm of deeply connected Plant Healers, it is more often referred to as a field, community, or even tribe, and seldom as what is perhaps most accurate: a "family." The most common definition of family is a group of people related to one another by blood or marriage. For some, mere mention of the word immediately brings out warm and fuzzy feelings as thoughts of beloved mates, children and other close relatives joyously come to mind. There are often pleasant associations as well as comforting personal memories, fusing with a greater cultural nostalgia for the senses of security, trust, support and alliance that family used to represent.

There are others, of course, whose formative experience of nuclear family was largely dysfunctional, with abusive or absent parents, or whose own attempts at marriage and child rearing were disappointing or traumatic. We may have never felt like we truly fit in, never had a family we could genuinely identify with and count on, an intimate circle of support, or a group that we knew in our hearts we belonged to.

Ahh, but we do belong, even the most independent or alienated, isolated or sidelined, shy or misfit of us! We are by virtue of our callings, our caring about others, our knowledge and skills, and our faithful love for the plants, each a part of a family of fellow herbal-hearted beings.

Like an extended family in ancient times, today's Plant Healers share many of the same needs and knowings, a common language and terminology, common mythology and iconography, similar sensibilities, attractions to and estimations of beauty, resonant curiosities and sense of wonder, related concerns, and intentions to help heal others and this planet.

Wherever we are situated, anywhere on the globe, we are motivated by a desire to ease suffering and mend what is torn asunder, we're subject to a class of threats from increasing regulation of plant medicine to corporate hegemony, as well as our own inflexible beliefs or faulty assumptions.

Likewise, the work we all do is tightly related, whether it be assisting the healthcare of our kids or our neighborhood, growing medicinal plants in our backyard garden, making medicines in our kitchen, selling our own herbal products, operating an apothecary, teaching and writing about herbalism, or actively conserving the herbs and their vital habitats.

If someone in this Plant Healer family is ill, or loses someone close to them, we all worry, bless, and often offer our emotional support, donations or other help. If someone's apothecary is shut down by regulators, or the name of their little neighborhood business appropriated by uncaring *corporados*, we do not need to have ever met them to recoil in empathetic response. When we see a posting announcing another child born amongst us, we can't help but celebrate the arrival of little Juniper or Sage. We are stirred to do what we can for pop-up herbal clinics after local disasters, and to sponsor activists protecting and re-wilding plant habitat. Congratulations are in order, whenever we hear about the launching of a community centered clinic or home-based herbal school, and we tend to be demonstrably sentimental over the hanging of a freshly painted sign above a now open door.

For the folk herbalist – the beginner making their first medicines on a plant strewn kitchen counter, the cultivator of herbal gardens, the humble enthusiast of all things green – it can be a family that's more supportive than our own blood relatives, the place where all can be their herb focused selves no matter how different or strange they might think themselves. It where we go to be seen for who we really are, and to express our concerns and obsession and hopes without fear of being dismissed or attacked.

We are all "family healthcare providers," providing whatever useful and accurate healing information we are able to regardless of how much we still do not know, taking care of clients and neighbors the way we might care for our parents and offspring, and drawing from and giving back to the family of Plant Healers that are each an integral, evolving, giving and sustaining part of.

In times of social, political and environmental dis-ease, when there is so much to feel alienated, affronted, or even threatened by, it is wondrously comforting and empowering to know there are others of our ilk, sisters and brothers of compassion, fellow apprentices to the plants and relatives of the wild, with similar and allied purposes. When we are questioning or feeling alone, we need only reach out for the understanding, counsel and encouragement of other members of this family, from towns and cities far and wide. When possible, we form lasting partnerships, alliances, and the most essential connections. At special times we may come together under a common tent of stars to meet in person, learn and laugh together in a familial ritual of Good Medicine Confluences.

When identifying the herbs we use, we pay attention to its taxonomic rankings. Above Genus and below Order are the plant Families (that part of the scientific names usually ending in-*aceae*). We share a family in a similar way, Plant Healer*aceae*, a community that is like a gathering of diverse songs for a vital concert, together carrying forth diverse traditions, perspective, personal preferences and expressions of the healing practice, with our different ways and times of sprouting, a nearly infinite variety of rainbow hued blossoms, and yet all sharing a common vine of values and purpose… you and we, inextricably entwined at the roots.

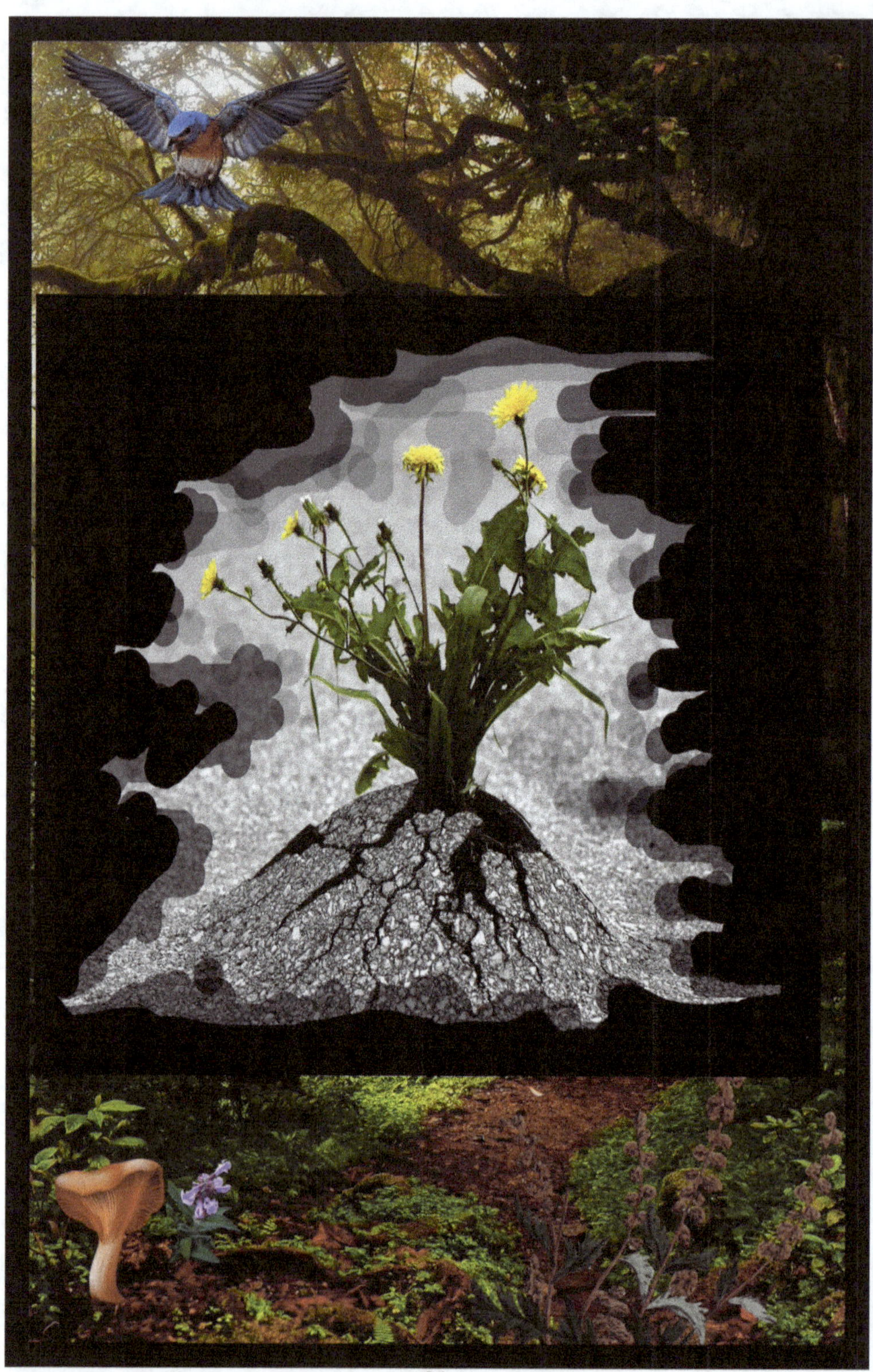

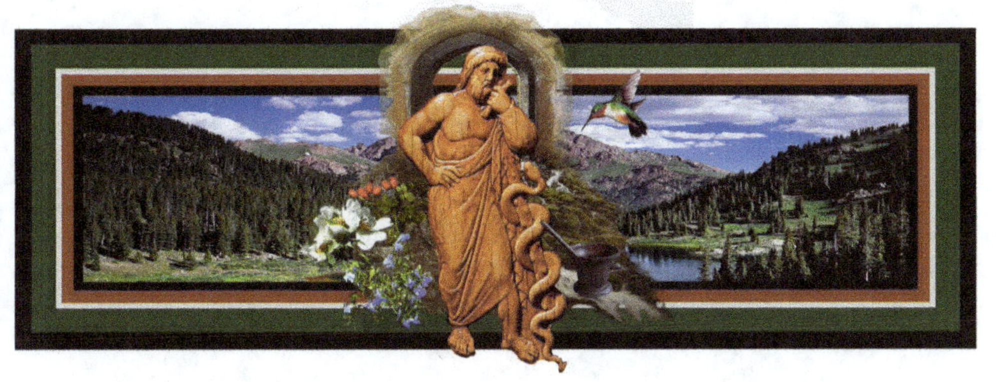

OUR DANDELION
RESURGENCE

Picture for a moment, if you will, the concrete covering much of any city. Now imagine a small crack somewhere in it, wrested open by the heaving breathing, freeze and thaw of a living earth intolerant of stasis and control. Picture, too, the vibrant green expression of the vital life force as it sinuously wriggles and forces its way upwards towards the sun, resplendent with its disorderly leaves, it's shameless yellow flower-heads unbowed and un-saddened: the proverbial outlaw Dandelion!

We healers, herbalists and culture-shifters can be a lot like Dandelions and other insistent and persistent plants – a lot like them in our finding ways to sprout in even the most sterile of environs, in our promotion of diversity, in our penetration of the supposedly impenetrable, in our resistance to restraint… and we're a lot like them in our seeking and discovering of openings and opportunities that allow both our true natures and nature's healing ways to blossom again.

Like the Dandelion, the plant healer is by nature an agent of both restoration and a great enlivening, as well as a symbol of strong if gentle persistence in the face of eras of increased repression, exclusion, distraction or neglect. Plant Healers have at times joined Dandelions in being demeaned by society, and denigrated like weeds.

Most importantly, the encroaching concrete that the Dandelion suffers under, bedevils herbalists as well – in the form of not only oppressive regulation and restrictions, but also our own traditions and beliefs whenever they limit our evolution and innovation. It's manifest in official systems and biases that can make folks with any level of knowledge and expertise feel insufficient, unworthy, excluded or trivialized... and in that crusting slurry of self doubt that can wash over us and cement us to the floor.

Like the dandelion, herbalism and alternative culture prospers, gestates and spreads surreptitiously whenever suppressed, feeling right at home in the "underground." Neither walls nor borders can restrain it. If there be but a single fissure anywhere in that which holds it down, it is through this opening that our practices will surge forth into the light of day once more.

Dissed as a "weed" by a majority of citizens, poisoned with herbicides, or ignominiously yanked from the ground by even some lovers of gardens, the Dandelion nonetheless continues to not only persist but flourish.

This plant serves us as both a symbol and an agent of insistent self determination in the face of conformity and control, expressions of a natural resurgent vitality in creative resistance to the unhealthy ways and stultifying sameness of the dominant paradigm. It is medicine for the liver, medicine for the ecosystem, and medicine for our ways of perceiving ourselves and our role in this world and work. Dandelion resurgence. Dandelion healing. Dandelion delight.

And like the Dandelion, the plant healer's practice is itself a living thing, as caring as the most sentient creature, while also being plant-like in its powers of resilience, resumption, and regeneration.

Again and again folk herbalism has quieted and receded of its own accord, or been systematically repressed.   It's been alternately embraced. and dissed. In its Autumns and Winters, it draws into itself. Its roots continue to grow, but its vines rest from their earlier wrangling, its leaves fallen or hung snow-bent in contemplation. In its Springs and Summers, new growth is awakened, and new sprouts burst forth from hungering seeds.

Every bit as important as a return to our roots is for all of us – is the reclaiming of herbalism's intrinsic spirit and essential organic nature, its informality and egalitarianism, social consciousness and courageous response. Ours is a remembering of the original feelings and motivations that have always inspired this work with medicinal plants. And ours is a surging forward to self empowerment and grass roots action, mated with the reawakening of the curiosity, excitement, and giddy pleasures of this healing work.

What we are doing together is fostering and fueling a resurgence of empowered herbalism. Our resurgence is made up of strong passions and caring insistence, wild-heartedness and nonconformity, awareness and action, love and devotion that – *just like the health-full outlaw Dandelion –* busts through even the hardest of concrete.

Trust me — we have within us the Dandelion's wondrous weedy power that nothing can ever keep down. And no one can ever hold us back from this needed healing dance.

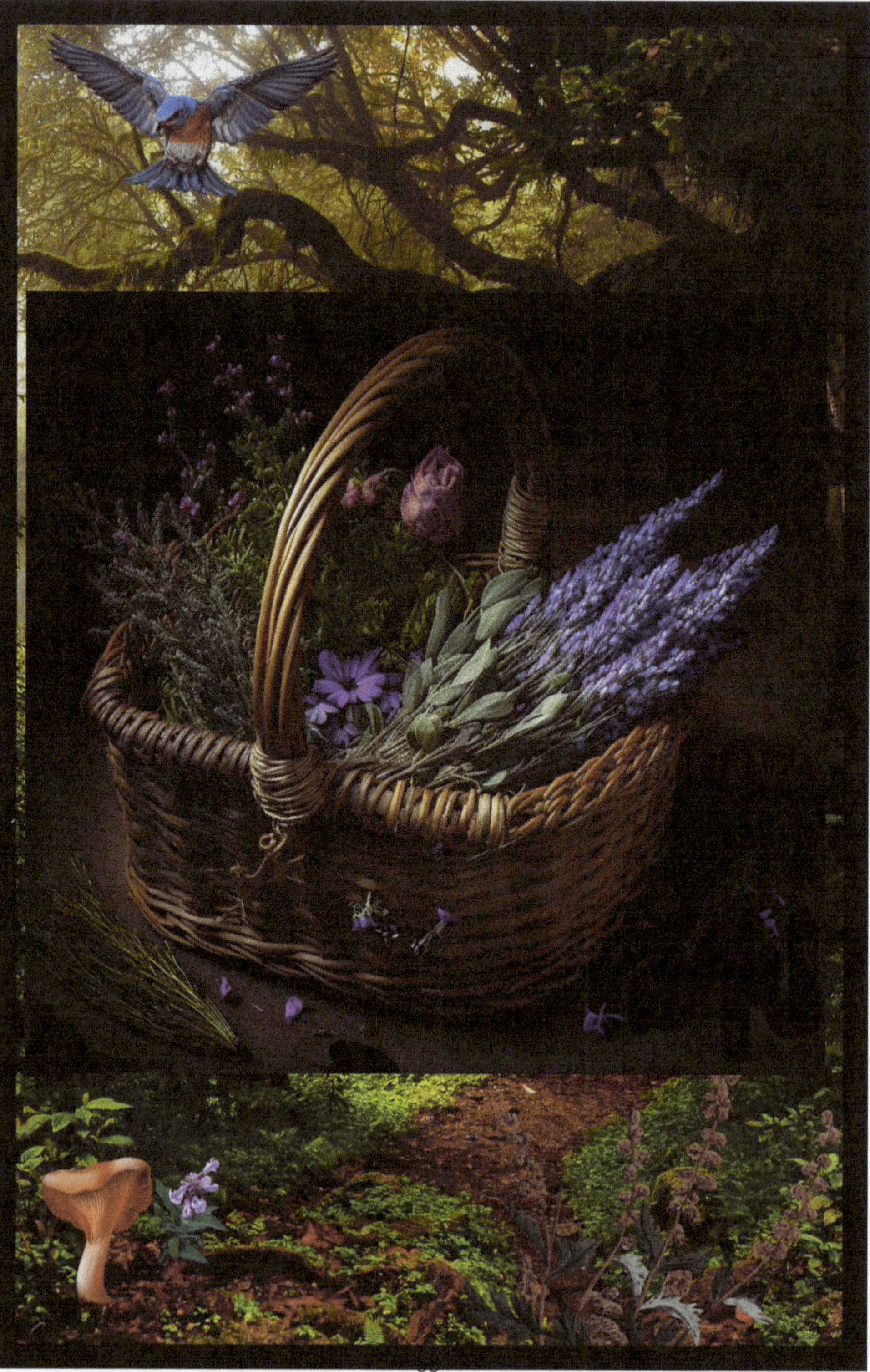

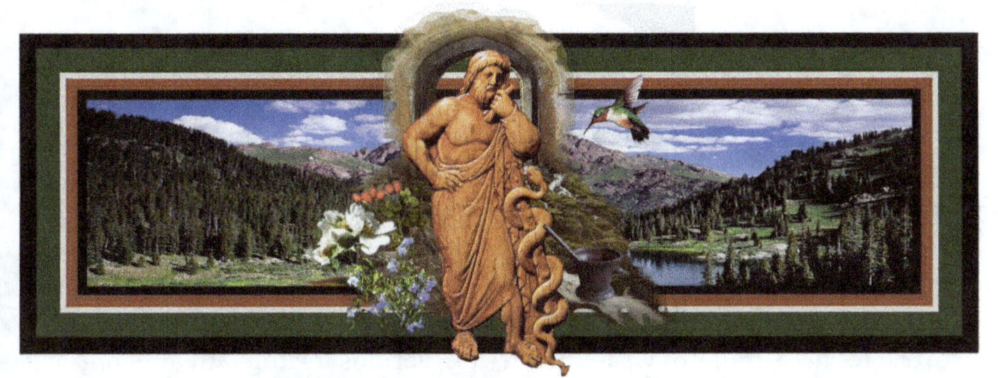

20 WAYS
TO ROYALLY FUCK UP
YOUR HERBAL PRACTICE

We've previously talked about ten ways to be the very best herbalist that you can be, along with ten moral characteristics of a caring natural healer. Equally useful is our recognition of the following twenty ways to royally fuck up what could otherwise be a lifelong, super effective, and completely satisfying practice.

So, 20 ways to blow it…. let's roll:

1. Firstly, we screw up when we recommend herbs and protocols based just on their usual widely known uses, without factoring in each person's individual nature, constitutional type, metabolism, lifestyle, health history, and health goals.

2. We are mess up by emphasizing rare, exotic, imported, or trending herbs over local, proliferate, or seldom written about plant medicines. And by ignoring local herbal corollaries and possible effective substitutes.

3. We mess up by treating physical, bodily health conditions without also taking into account mental health, attitude, diet, exercise, lifestyle, receptivity and compliance.

89

4. We error whenever we treat with herbs *only*, without also considering other potentially helpful modalities and methods to at least recommend trying in conjunction with plant medicines — for example, things like: tonifying mushrooms, vitamin replenishment, removing certain aggravating food types, emotional therapy, physical therapy, hydrotherapy, acupuncture, and dedicated time in the healing outdoors.

5. We are blowing it whenever we forget to record the case studies of those we try to help, fail to write down the various factors, treatments and outcomes — or don't take the time to look for patterns indicating other possible courses of action to follow in the future.

6. We fuck up by working mainly with processed components and isolates, without also taking into account the value of starting with whole plants and taking advantage of their particular symphonic balance of different chemicals and effects.

7. We mess up by dissing new scientific research as all being lies foisted on us by big business spin-masters, when we should be critically assessing and often integrating and utilizing new discoveries, data, and understandings.

8. Or we blow it doing exactly the opposite, imagining that research is ever truly unbiased, or else by accepting its conclusions at face value.

9. We can screw up by either placing too little importance on plant biochemistry, energetics and actions, or else, by placing too much!

10. By dissing the value of "book learning," or conversely, by not putting enough stock in the importance of our gaining personal experience.

11. By thinking that the reason medicinal plants exist on this planet is for human uses rather than firs and foremost being here for themselves and their communities, or that it is a plant's destiny or desire to be cut down or pulled up.

12. By accepting the sacrifice of plants' lives and the aid that they provide without giving back to them through means like thankfulness, seed dispersal and cultivation, or crucial habitat protection.

13. By not putting enough time into herbal studies, or into gaining actual experience.

14. Or conversely, by giving so much time to an herbal business that you consequently neglect yourself, neglect your other priorities, or end up distanced from the vital passion and excitement of working with plants.

15. By beginning to think that you know all you need to about some plant or condition, or acting as if there's no valuable new information to be learned.

16. We mess up by failing to experiment, to use a well known herb for some as yet unheard of application, to explore new formulations, or to test out your insights and hunches.

17. By failing to take chances, such as recommending herbs for conditions conventionally treated using pharmaceuticals, such as moving to a new location that better serves your needs, practice or spirit... or quitting an unsatisfying job to focus on a coveted herbal career or start a plant hearted business.

18. We blow it by measuring our worth by our income or popularity, instead of by the compassion of our intentions and the actual evident effects that our healing practices and efforts have.

19. We blow it by imagining that we do not know enough about herbs to dare to try and help people, that we don't have what it takes to ever be good enough, or that our contributions aren't valuable just because there are other practitioners who are more informed or have practiced longer. By being too self demeaning, doubtful or afraid to give our lives whole heartedly to what we love most and to fully live our dreams.

20. And finally, forgetting to have fun can fuck things up as much as anything else. The serious business of healing illnesses possibly saving lives can lead to exhaustion or burnout without our deliberate focused efforts on the Plant Healer's pleasures, on the sensory and sensual rewards of working with these amazing green being, and on actively and fully enjoying what we dedicate ourselves to... and we can do this caring work all the better, and sustain it for far longer, if we also make sure to have a helluva good time while we're at it!

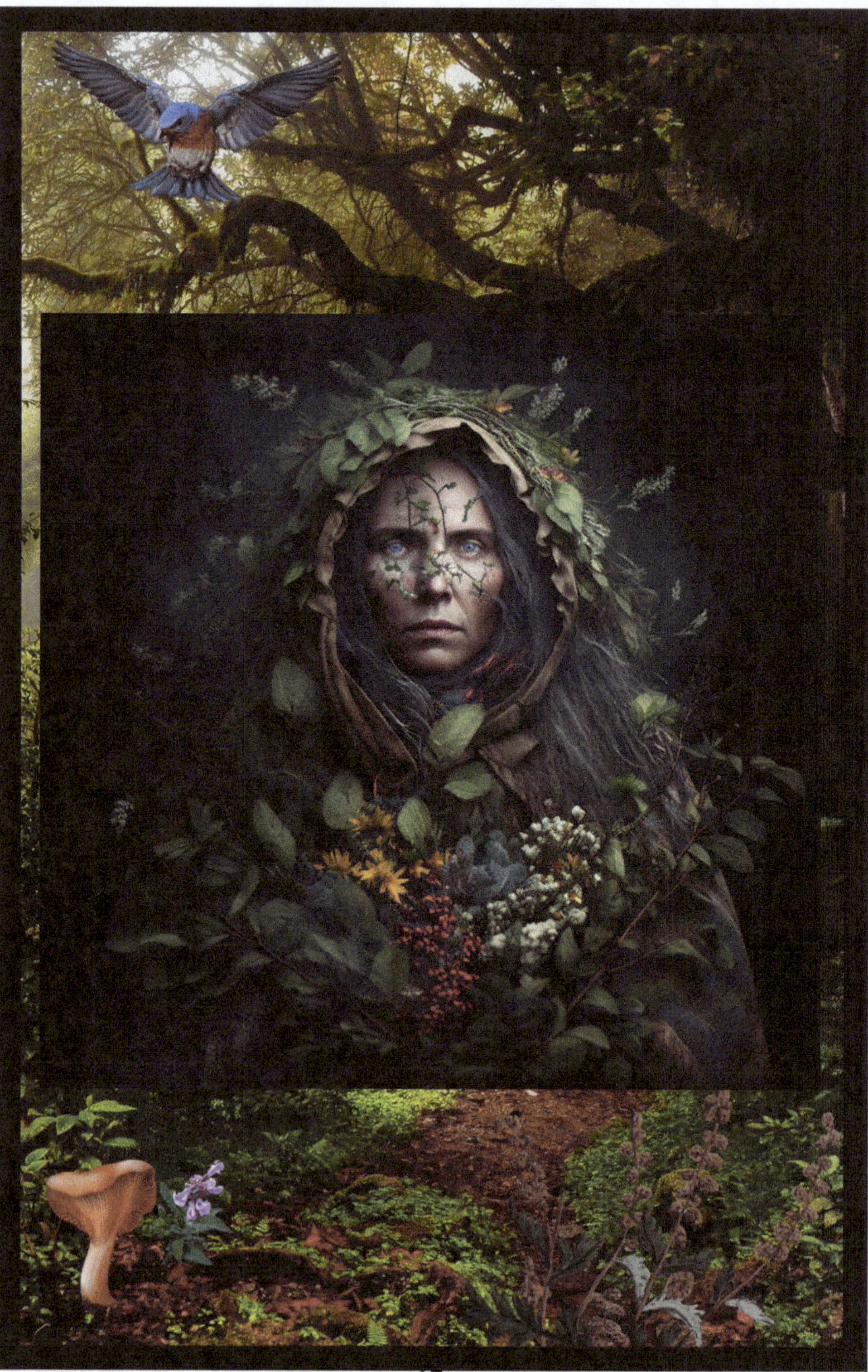

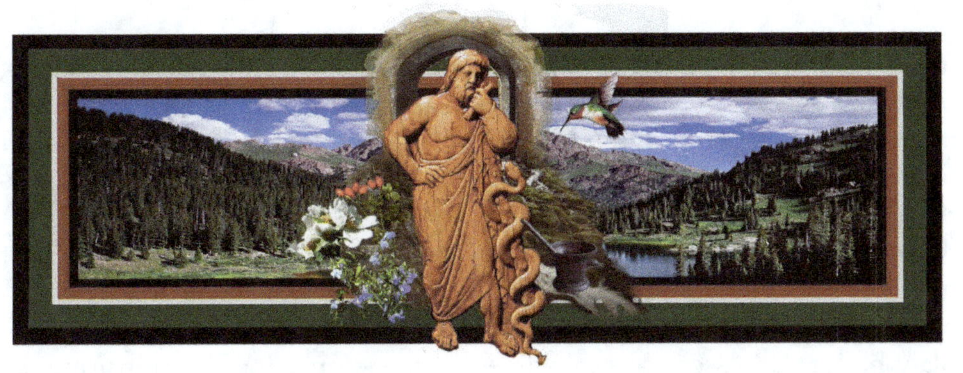

THE NATURE
IN NATURAL HEALING

In an age when commercial herbal remedies are found on every grocery store's shelves, and almost every kind of alternative therapy can be found in town, it can be all too easy to forget what the "natural" in "natural healing" really means — and too easy to lose sight of the natural world from which all medicinal plants arise, the nature that without which humanity cannot survive.

Too often nature gets portrayed as something separate from us, a threatening place outside the protective boundaries of civilization, when what it really is is our original and essential home! Nature is *us* at our most authentic, embodied, and proactive. Nature is where we get grounded and oriented, where we can find and gather the healing herbs we need. It's where we encounter our authentic, most sentient selves, where we are are made aware of our most meaningful purpose and ideal individual roles, the place where we're presented with the inspiration and essential lessons that we need.

Health itself is a natural state, with our bodies naturally working to protect and restore themselves, and usually the most helpful and least harmful treatments come from natural plant medicines and the therapeutic effects of living a more natural life.

Indeed, the human body functions as an ecosystem, as a dynamic balancing of various energetic systems and physiological functions, as an aggregate of interrelated, interactive and ultimately interdependent parts. The study and tending of that bodily whole, is what I call an "ecology of healing." It leads the thoughtful plant healer to take a wholistic, ecosystems approach – thinking of and treating human beings as interconnected systems of qualities and processes, rather than focusing mainly on some isolated organ or symptom. As you probably know, one of the most effective ways that the plant healer addresses physical ailments is by supporting and nurturing the body overall.

I can give you a few tips for helping keep nature at the heart of our natural healing practice:

• Try working more with whole and even fresh plants.

• When you look at even herbal capsules and preparations, see them as the herbs they are made from. Never put it out of your mind that the best medicines we use are *plants*, not just products or constituents but actual physical beings, their essence and spirit, energy and actions.

• Train yourself to recognize the patterns of causes and actions, study the ways in which things interrelate and interact — including human bodies and environments, organs and systems, physical and emotional processes.

• Instead of mainly working with the most popularly consumed or exotic imported species, try local corollaries, and introduce more common and weedy herbs.

• Take regular plant walks, in which you pay special attention to the different botanical species along your sidewalks, in your parks, and in the closest forests to where you live.

• Find time for some monthly wildcrafting, taking trips into wild public lands whenever you can, and otherwise gathering herbs from urban lots and suburban hills. Note what plants are scarce or hurting, and only take from places where they are plentiful.

• Hold the plants not just in hand but in heart. Consciously feed and grow an ever evolving relationship with them that is intensely personal, intimate, emotional, even spiritual and cellular!

• Sense the plants' millions of years of accumulated wisdom, the different multi-faceted lessons that each species has to offer, and ways in which they can be incredible examples and role models to us.

• Give back to the plants you use in some direct, tangible, personal way such as planting a garden of scarce or endangered herb species, setting aside part of your yard for the reintroduction of wild native plants, working to protect threatened habit in your region, spreading prudently selected seeds widely in joyous acts of what I am silly enough to call "unauthorized public plantings."

• Consider and assess the individual natures of your clients and anyone else you hope to help. Take into account their natural constitutions when considering what to treat them with.

• Advise clients on the healthy effects of time outside, of sun on our skin, sexuality, forest bathing, immersion in cold streams, natural foods and fermentation, and strenuous exercise.

• You can improve your herbal work, increase your discoveries and realizations, and experience more of its rewards by constantly developing your innate, natural characteristics — such as your creature curiosity and awakened physical senses. Your primordial instincts and inexplicable intuition. Your urge to explore the unknown, and your courage to test all limits and bounds. The passion that you naturally put into the things you do, whenever you give full agency *to natural you.*

It is the nature of healing that it attracts folks like yourself — some of the most deeply feeling, deeply caring, visionary, revolutionary, and *effective* of health providers.

It is in your own nature to choose this loving work.

And there can be no natural healing without nature.

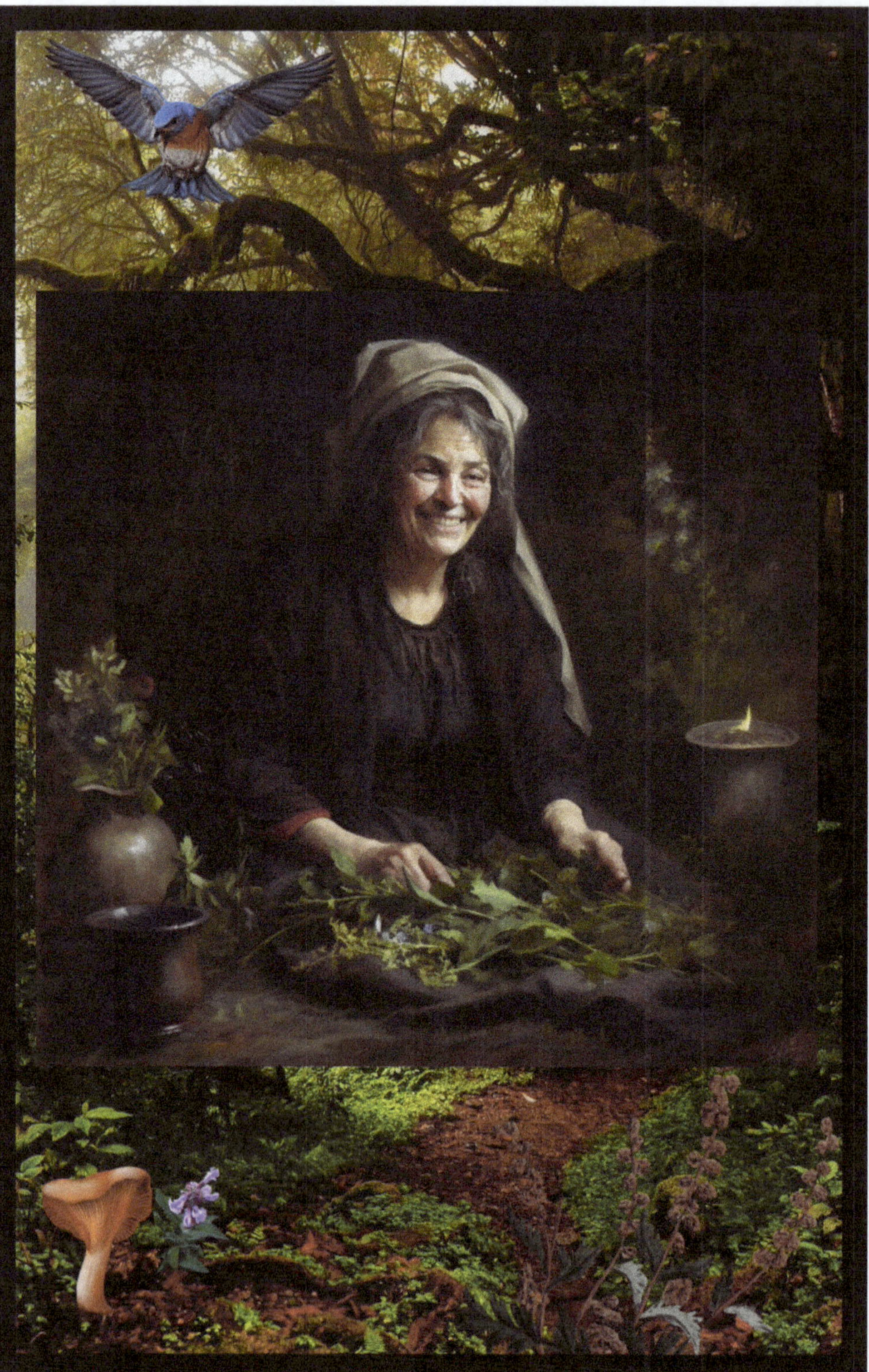

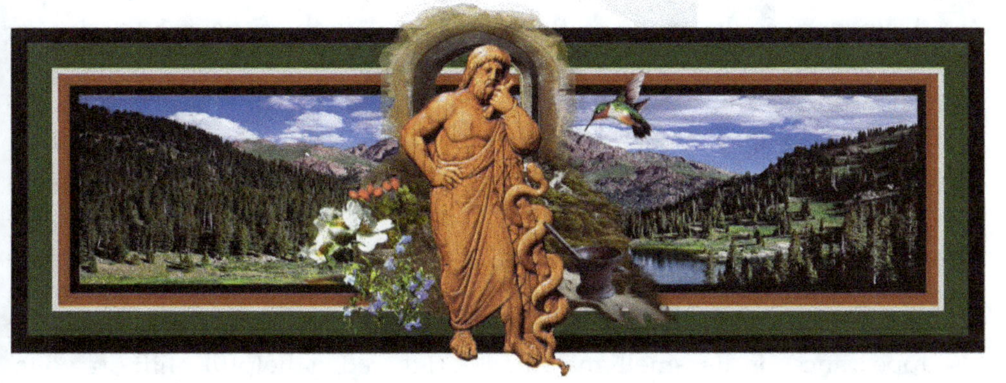

YOUR PERSONAL HERBAL ALLY
THE ONE PLANT THAT WILL
TEACH & SERVE YOU BEST

I find that herbal practitioners and wildcrafters, gardeners and gourmands, botanical artists and nature lovers, are often deeply in love with the wondrous beauty and amazing effects of plants in general. If asked about our favorites, it may be that we admire so many that it becomes hard to narrow it down to just a few. There is for each of us, however, most likely a single, particular green being that will either hold special significance or play a remarkable part in our unfolding lives.

Similar to what's called someone's animal "familiar," "totem" or "guide," that plant ally might be for you an ancient towering Redwood or maybe a gnarly limbed Cedar that you always go to sit beneath for counsel and solace. Your special plant may serve as a symbol, or as an example, or even as a role model — like a lowland Oak whose strength and fortitude you strive to embody, or maybe the prickly Wild Rose that you identify with so much, that exemplary bramble that no weed whacker or paver can ever hold down! Your ally could have roots or petals that you make sure to carry with you wherever you go, nestled inside a deer hide medicine bag. Or you may be known for decorating your home, your computer or your clothing with its evocative leafen image.

Its distinction could be a matter of timing, with it having made an unexpected appearance, revealing itself to you during a pivotal moment of transition or in a time of great need. Perhaps you've noticed it right there close after a painful breakup, or on the day a child is born, or while celebrating a hard earned accomplishment or milestone event. Your special plant may have proven to be a crucial catalyst or an important facilitator. It might trigger a shared experience that brings you and your sweetheart closer together, or perhaps develop into the botanical emblem of some alliance or cause that you've pledged yourself to. More often, its company, its appearance or its smell may have triggered a helpful shift in your thinking, or maybe has propelled the flow of new ideas, or provided some realization that's brought you much needed peace.

For those of you that are herbalists, your special plant is likely defined by its healing effects. You might be walking a park path when a certain weed seems to call for your attention, beckoning with its branches in the evening winds. You may not be able to resist a sniff and a taste, and after looking it up in your plant identification books it might turn out to be exactly the medicine you most need to help a friend or client. You could have retreated atop a sunlit hill, trying to calm and gather yourself after weeks of unsuccessfully treating some bedeviling health problem of your own — only to discover that you sat down among the exact kinds of flowers that will end up healing you. Your special ally could even be that one medicinal herb that saved your life when you couldn't find anything else that could help.

It may a plant that you've yet to be introduced to, or on the other hand, it could be one that you've been familiar with for years but are only just now coming to really hear, embrace, learn from and connect with. Seek out and then feel out plants that seem to convey the deepest or most urgent meaning. And look again at the many plants you already work with or walk amongst, consider how they relate to you and your purposes, what they seem to symbolize, the songs they seem to sing, the knowing they share, the responses they suggest, the hopes and dreams they excite.

It's not just a species that you find interesting or beautiful. Rather, it's an instrumental and irreplaceable *significator* — extremely relevant, inevitably influential, utilizable, unforgettable. Once you're sure of yours, celebrate *fergawdsake!* Take inspiration from it as needed, in the best of times and in the most difficult or perplexing of situations, every busy day and restful night. It is your truth teller and teacher, your helper and light bearer, your agent and icon, and your friend… your own personal herbal ally.

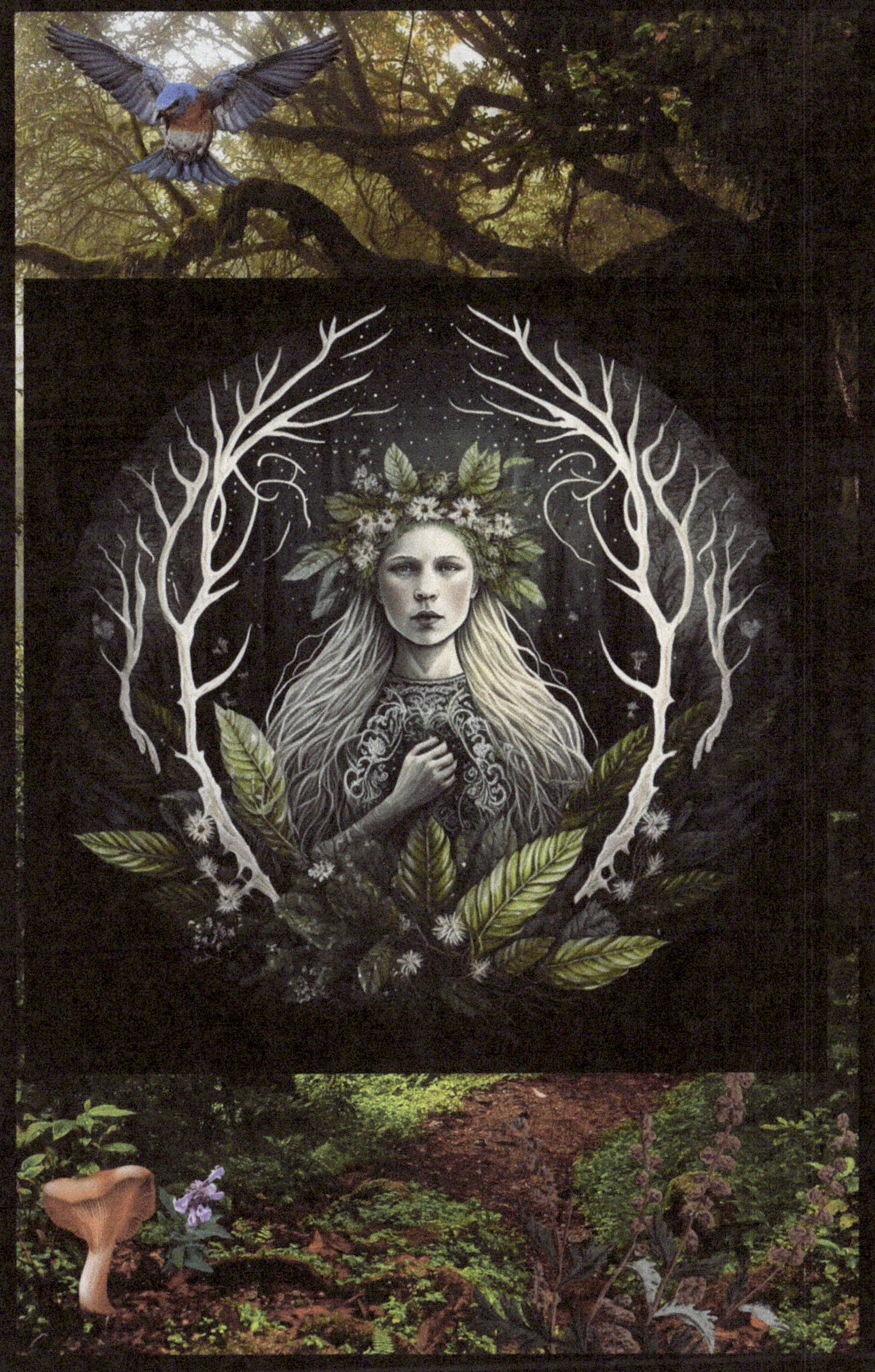

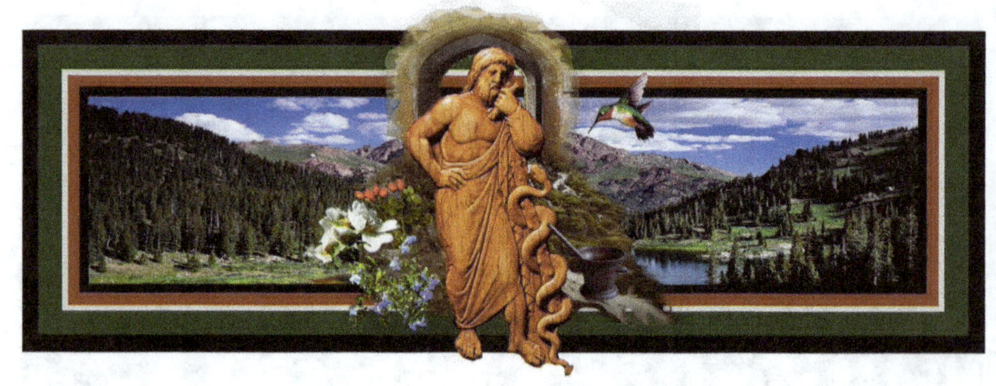

An Herbal Liturgy

The Enlightenment, Spirituality & Magic of The Healing Arts

There can be no denying that folk herbalism and most natural healing practices are rooted in a spiritual and magical sensibility, not some rigid dogma or blind belief, but a bone-deep knowing that life is animated not just by a swirling of neurons and recombining chemicals, but by an inner, inherent force or spirit. No amount of science or reason can overshadow the awesomeness of birth, the improbability and near miraculousness of wounds closing over and disappearing within days and before our very eyes. Not even the most advanced understanding of plant biochemistry, energetics and actions can ever take away from the seeming magic of herbs visibly relieving, mending and restoring us.   Even the brevity of our finite lifespans can contribute to our spiritual awakening to life's ebb and flow, its subsiding and deconstructing, its reemergence and its surges, its healings and its repairs.

Sure, we need knowledge as much as hope, experience and experimentation as much as faith, but research, information and skills are most useful when fueled and propelled by strong feelings of interconnection and oneness, of the sacred, the magical, and the wondrous.

Whether walking to my remote river canyon home, gathering wild herbs from beside the trail, or working with the tinctures and salves that they provide — everything seems to me somehow alive, inspirited and energized. And indeed, it is: Spirit in the myriad plants and animals, and in the unfolding lessons of terrestrial Gaia. Spirit vibrating within volcanic rocks, glowing in the light of a setting sun. Spirit in a plant's taste and scent, in sensuality and struggle, in both our challenges and our fun. Spirit in the life giving river, and in the giddy intercourse of evolving life forms. Spirit in a hopeful child's face. Spirit in the hearts and deeds of they who serve the processes and aims of truth, of place, of healing and love. Spirit doing the seemingly impossible, emboldening the planting of roots in what is an always shifting shore, inspiring us to give ourselves to the mission of making things better in the face of what may look like overwhelming challenges. Spirit tracing its own movements in a lover's grazing touch or the designs drawn by windblown weeds in the riverbank sand, and spirit empowering every healer's helpful hand.

The root meaning of the word "spirit" is "breath:" a clear volume of energy that one can best feel when it moves, alerts, prods or pushes, seduces or agitates. Spirituality, then, can be understood as an act of tireless respiration and is thus reciprocal, rhythmically taking in and giving back in equal measure. But it isn't so much the ways that we think about spirit, as it is the ways in which we embody its processes and its grace, practice its magical arts, own and then pass on its vital lessons. It is both committed and proactive, and no matter what its form or container it requires our direct experiencing, our direct relationship, and our utilization. This often begins with a growing awareness that we cannot ignore, and with levels of distraction and dishonor that we can no longer tolerate. It involves conscious, mystical connection, interdependence and interpenetration, expanding empathy and heightened sensation, contact and contracts with the inspirited land and its creatures and plants, its vibrational entities and insistent inspiriteurs. A spiritual life doesn't denigrate or deny desirous existence. Its hungers, disappointments and pleasures are as catalysts accelerating our manifestation, transformation and growth.

This healer's spirituality is an assignment that we sign up for again and again, each and every moment — an impeccable dance that we do, a set of promises that we keep. It is compassion and caring fully given. It's life fully lived... and our most meaningful purpose fulfilled.

Awakening to the magic can feel both transformative and blissful, a state of self-realization and intense mindfulness sometimes referred to as "satori," "samadhi" or "enlightenment." Contrary to what you may have been told, this state of being is not about transcending matter or flesh, but rather, it's about our re-immersion in the depth and breadth of embodied reality: deep seeing, deep tasting and smelling, deeply dreaming, manifesting, and actualizing…. reaching out and touching the greater universe through this immediate world that is not so much "ours" as it is "us."

"We must remember the chemical connections between our cells and the stars, between the beginning and now. We must remember and reactivate the primal consciousness of oneness between all living things. We must return to that time, in our genetic memory, in our dreams, when we were one species born to live together on Earth as her magic children."
—Barbara Mor

Our personal spirituality and all that we intuit and learn, has got to be embodied, applied and maximized if we're to either reap the full benefits or effectively help this world. You Plant Healers are like blessed participants in the dance of embodied spirit, as dreamers and doers, as caregivers and praise givers. Your optimum practice is one that inspires and invokes awareness, reconnection, and right action. As from a place of fear and forgetting, you arise, revealed to be a responsible celebrant of amazing existence, as an agent of incomprehensible process, as the Druid priests and priestesses guarding and tending the sacred oaken groves, and as playmates and vehicles for omnipresent spirit. Together we co-create a more healthy reality, not as indentured servants of magic or some deity's obedient soldiers, but as ecstatic organs and willful extensions of an inspirited organic whole.

Make no mistake about it, so-called enlightenment isn't figuring out all the answers, it's literally casting a light on the inner recesses of one's truth and being and mission. It's the powerful experience of conscious interconnectedness, the wordless timeless thrill of being thrust into full realization, relationship and responsibility, discovery and delight! Enlightenment doesn't exist to spare us any hard labors or difficult lessons. Instead, it thrusts us into the pulsing fabric of a rhythmic, patterned, and knowing universe.... and in this way, back into a most powerful and pleasurable version of our magical, purposeful and spiritual healer's lives.

We plant our caring seeds in heart and earth, and render our special medicines regardless of the given odds for success or fruition. We entirely invest ourselves into what is a liturgy of healing, with one immediate result being a more vibrant and bliss-filled experiencing and fulfilling of precious life — powerful visions, instrumental assignments, and the embracing of a personal healer's mission.... every day a testament to our glad participation in the magical and the miraculous, every moment witness to your devoted work of helping, and healing, and wholeness.

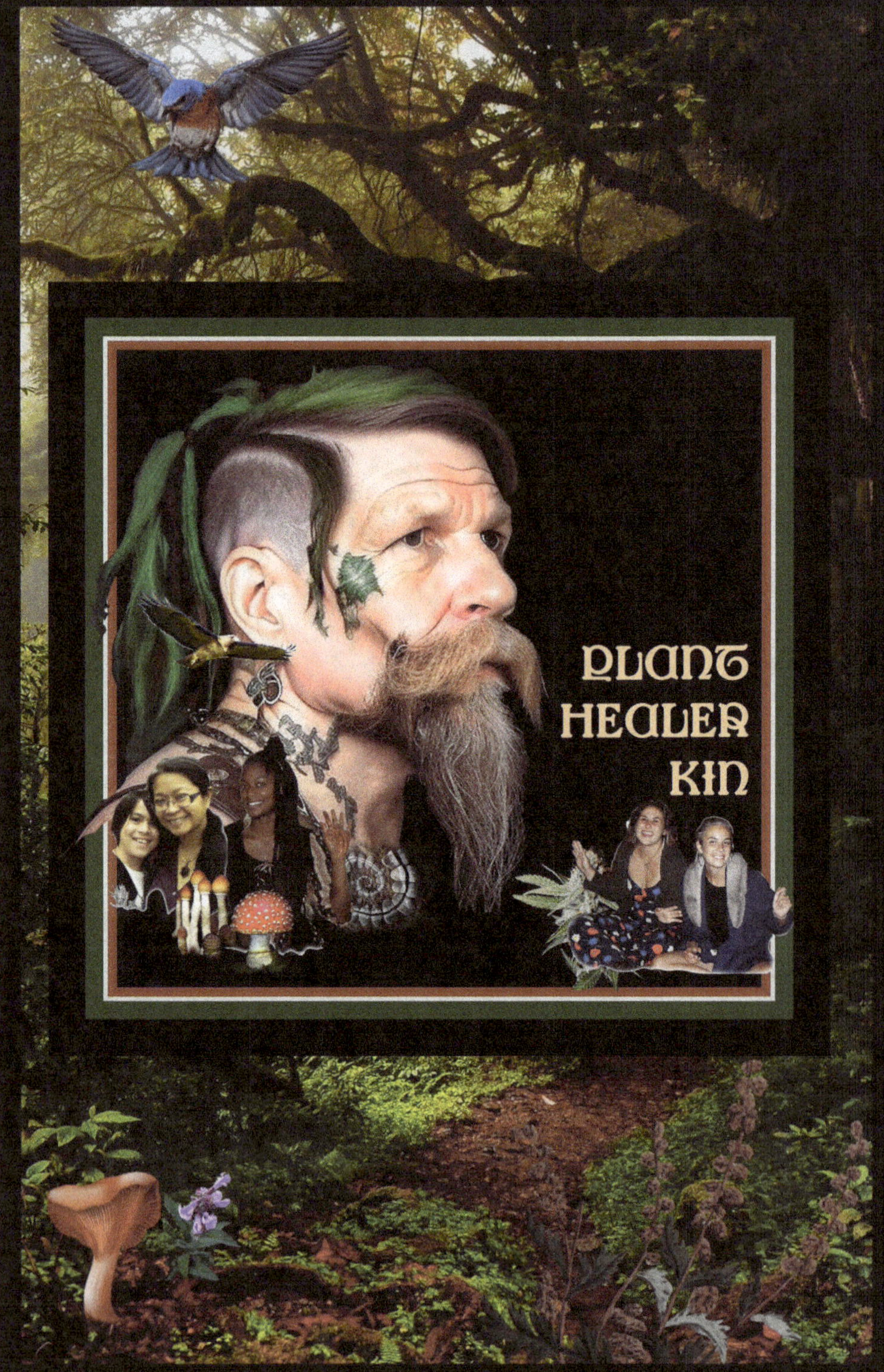
PLANT
HEALER
KIN

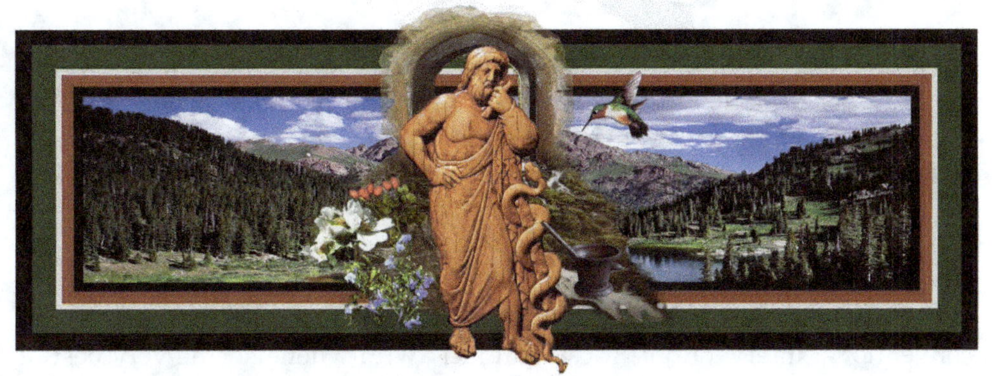

KNOWING WHAT YOU CAN
& CAN'T AFFECT

Anyone in any field can be outcome oriented, focused on a particular desired result, but for folks dedicated to ending suffering or saving lives this presents as not just an aim and intention but as a deeply felt and utterly urgent need. This is especially true for herbalists and healthcare providers, as well as for hands-on parents, culture shifters, justice and environmental advocates, reformers and activists of all kinds.

There are reasonable or at least limited expectations when it comes to most jobs and many different kinds of roles in life, while we tend to have arguably *unreasonable* goals when it comes to things that we have a deep emotional investment in — such as raising our children to become commendable and wholly fulfilled adults, things like putting an end to the constant wars around the world or slowing nuclear proliferation, protecting the mistreated peoples at the very margins of society, preserving climate balance or saving ecosystems from impending destruction... and such as our personal missions to help heal people's painful conditions and disabling diseases. And yeah, I find something uncommonly beautiful about even the most fruitless attempts to do the seemingly impossible.

Wish as we might, it's simply not in our power to banish all illness, right all wrongs, or end all wars. And yet, whether we're aware of it or not, in our hearts and our subconsciouses we often still expect ourselves to somehow or other come up with a successful plan — or therapy, or medicine — for all that ails, for all people, and the entire world!

We know damn well that we're not superheroes, and some of us may even go so far as to doubt the adequacy of our skills or the sufficiency of our knowledge, and yet we may feel like the many observable "mission impossibles" all weigh firmly on our shoulders.

Positive outcomes are rightfully central to most goals, and yet they're not always within our power to ensure. And while a Plant Healer understands that the progression of a disease can't always be halted with natural or even conventional interventions, it can still feel awful whenever the very best of our efforts fail to bring about a much hoped for result.

Look, we all want to be able to affect things. For many types of people, it's even in our very natures to want to crave a visible impact, and for some of us it can feel like a demanding imperative to make things better, to mend or to ease, to improve or to vitalize and maximize. The problem comes when we begin to measure ourselves primarily by what we're able affect or make happen, without taking fully into account how often there are problems or situations that nobody no matter how gifted or equipped can be sure to redirect, relieve or remedy.

A satisfying practice or mission to make people and things better, hinges in part on our both identifying and accepting that which we likely cannot affect, as well as a primary focus on all the good that we successfully accomplish day in and day out. Being aware of what we *can't* impact even with weeks or years of trying, can make it easier to figure out what things we actually *can* affect, and to start giving our energy to those projects and methods that most powerfully and demonstrably work.

A healer may understand that a certain disease cannot be gotten rid of completely with herbs, for example, and therefore give attention to strengthening a client's immune system and overall vitality, to reducing problematic symptoms, or even to possible non-botanical treatments. Similarly, an activist may not be able to stop the growth of a harmful industry, but we can possibly overturn an unjust state law or help protect a particular local forest from being clear cut, we can offer free services to the needy or plant endangered species in scarce habitat, or we can help to create educational content that slowly influences what's valued and guarded in a particular culture. And if public awareness campaigns or litigation fail, we might choose to give more of our time to protests or other measures and methods that are more immediately and more visibly impactful.

Of course, there are many, many worthy causes that can take years or even generations to bring to full fruition, and we may well need to push ahead on these issues regardless of any short term results — but the essential word here is "regardless." Where it becomes really unhealthy is when we delude ourselves, and give most of our thoughts, efforts and hours to plans with essentially zero possibility of success… and when we do so at the cost of having no energy left for impacting the world closer at hand, no time even for crucial self care.

The key to this dilemma, my friends, is for us to stop expecting total cures or permanent solutions, and instead, just to depend on ourselves making what we know has been and will surely continue to be a substantial, positive, and meaningful difference!

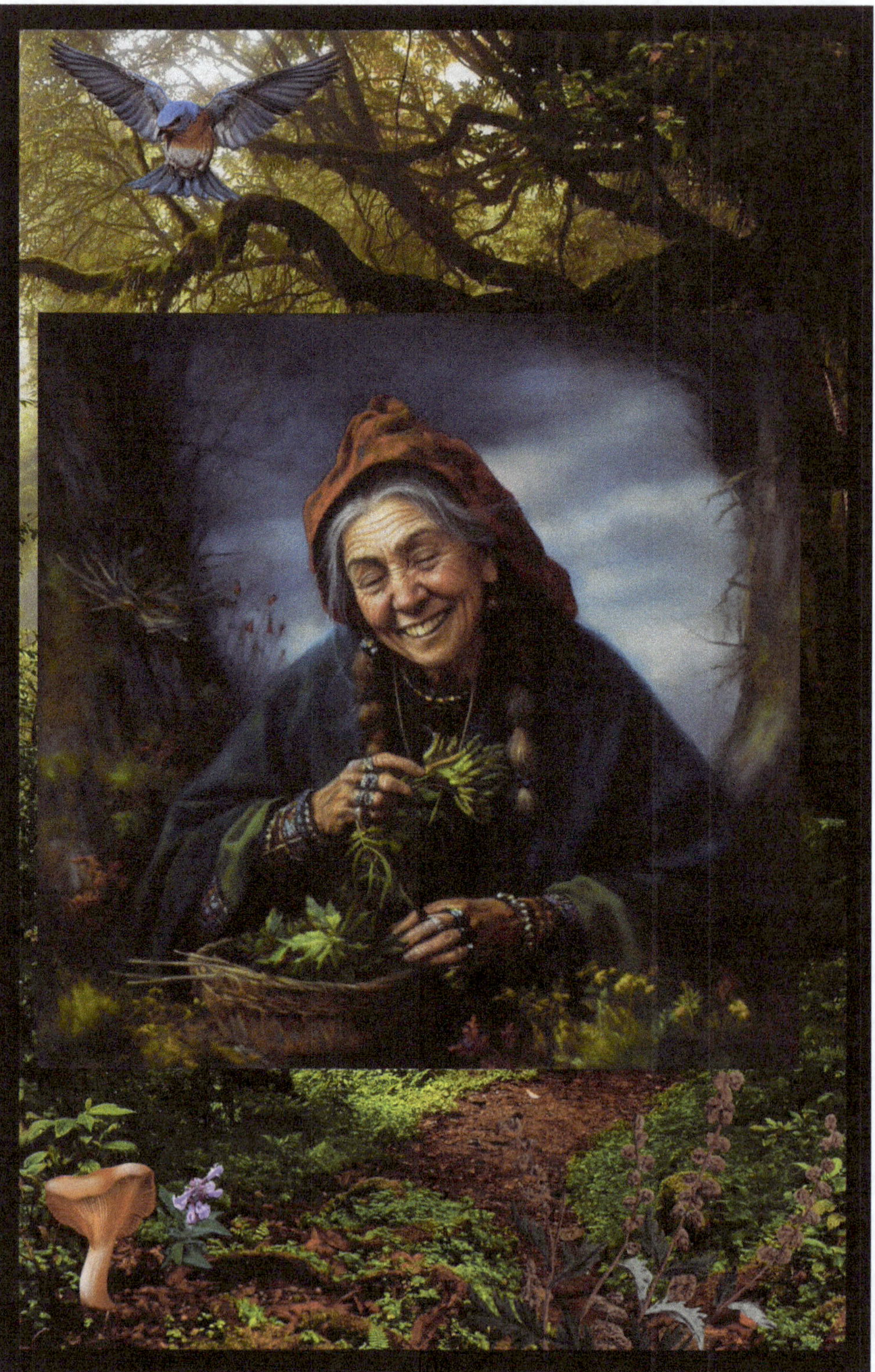

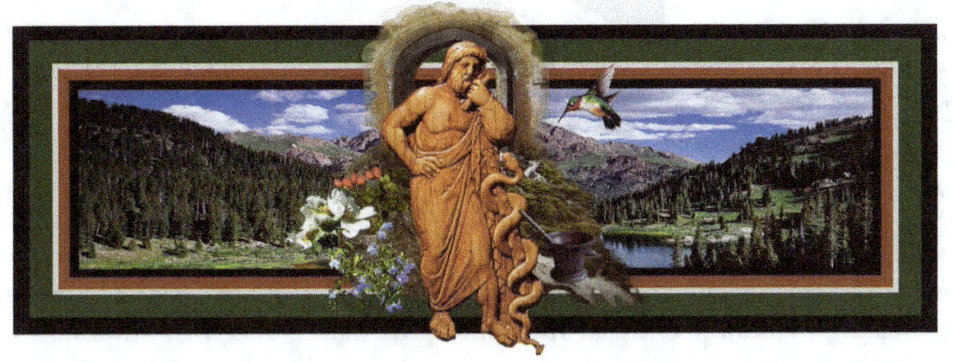

THE KINDNESS
OF HEALERS

One might think that herbalists would be indistinguishable from people with other interests and missions, but it simply isn't so. No matter what an herbalist's personality type, their passions and purpose tend to result in a particular set of characteristics that tend to make them identifiable, even when working alone with few or no fellow plant healers to ally with. The character of those attracted to some combination of serving the health of strangers, healing naturally, and studying and working with herbs are largely laudable, and often downright sweet and loving.

Sure, there are exceptions, maybe a small handful of holier-than-thous, and social media flareups and trollfests can bring out the frustrations in even the gentlest of souls… but the vast majority of herbalists are plant-hearted do-gooders doing some of the most underpaid and *kind* work on the planet.

kindness | ˈkīn(d)nəs | (n)
1. the quality of being friendly, generous, and considerate.

"Kind" is indeed the operative word here, should we be so silly as to try to define plant healers with any single term. But as you might assume, other "terms and conditions" do apply:

• Thoughtful, as in thinking about the needs and feelings of others, even of strangers. Thoughtful about wildcrafting common weedy species instead of harvesting rare or even endangered plants. Thoughtful about purchasing herbs from ethical businesses, and the impacts of their personal lifestyle and daily choices.

• Unselfish, in providing medicines and services to those in need at a low price, giving health advice suggestions to any who ask, sometimes launching or volunteering at free clinics for marginalized communities or rushing to help in post disaster situations such as after a destructive hurricane or home swallowing wildfire, often scraping together cash donations when someone they value is sick or in trouble.

• Compassionate, with deep consideration of the suffering of others, and with deep and demonstrable caring. Sympathetic, not in the sense of pitying ill or damaged people, but of relating harmoniously to another being's feelings, a correspondence, a caring chord struck on well tuned heartstrings. Empathic, meaning the understanding of and palpable sharing of feelings from joy to distress.

• Gentle, with a soft touch and a kind word. Hospitable, often with a personable or neighborly demeanor. Friendly, and generally forgiving of flaws. Loving, which is a necessary quality of the most effective herbal healers.

• And kind as in beneficent, a word originating in the Latin *bene facere*, meaning to *do good*. While someone may rightly plan to make a living with their products or practice, or hope for acceptance and recognition for their work, at their core is almost always an overriding desire, a calling, an obsessing with a mission of doing good: tending and mending, comforting and strengthening, empowering and equipping, beautifying and unifying, helping to make the world healthy and whole again.

For this reason, it pains me to ever say something cynical, satirical or acerbic that might possibly hurt a healer's feelings. Humor and irreverence are ever more vital now in these increasingly fractured and humorless times, but I am sensitive about what gets communicated and determined to avoid being even accidentally unkind to my extremely kindly kindred clan. It pains me even more, to witness any of you being disrespected or bullied, regardless of whether I agree there was reason or not.

The suffering that attends and follows an unkind remark or action, almost always results in a succession of traumas and dramas passed from one person to the next, a septic wave of unwellness radiating outwards and causing harms far beyond the place and moment. Similarly, the results of a kind gesture can be consequential, healing, and far reaching. An open minded dialogue creates the conditions for understanding if not agreement. Forgiveness of others opens a path for our forgiveness of ourselves, and means we can give more of our hours to kind accomplishment rather than to unkindly conflicts. Words of encouragement can unleash a flood of self-belief and healthy confidence, fuel creativity and make fulfillment more likely. Showing our appreciation through thoughtful gifts and acts, increases the chances that the person we are grateful to will feel good enough about it to increase their giving and doing for others. Helping restore wild habitat for the sake of the plants has the side benefit of resulting in more of its medicine being available to herbalists and thus their clients in the future.

Your kindness cannot be denied. Your thoughtfulness. Your caring. Your compassion and generosity. Your natural tendency, learned ability or determined quest to *make things better*. It's not clueless, not dorky, not fluffy, not a weakness. It is your strength, so there is really no reason to hide it or devalue it.

You are kind. And it is partly for this reason, that you *are our kind*.

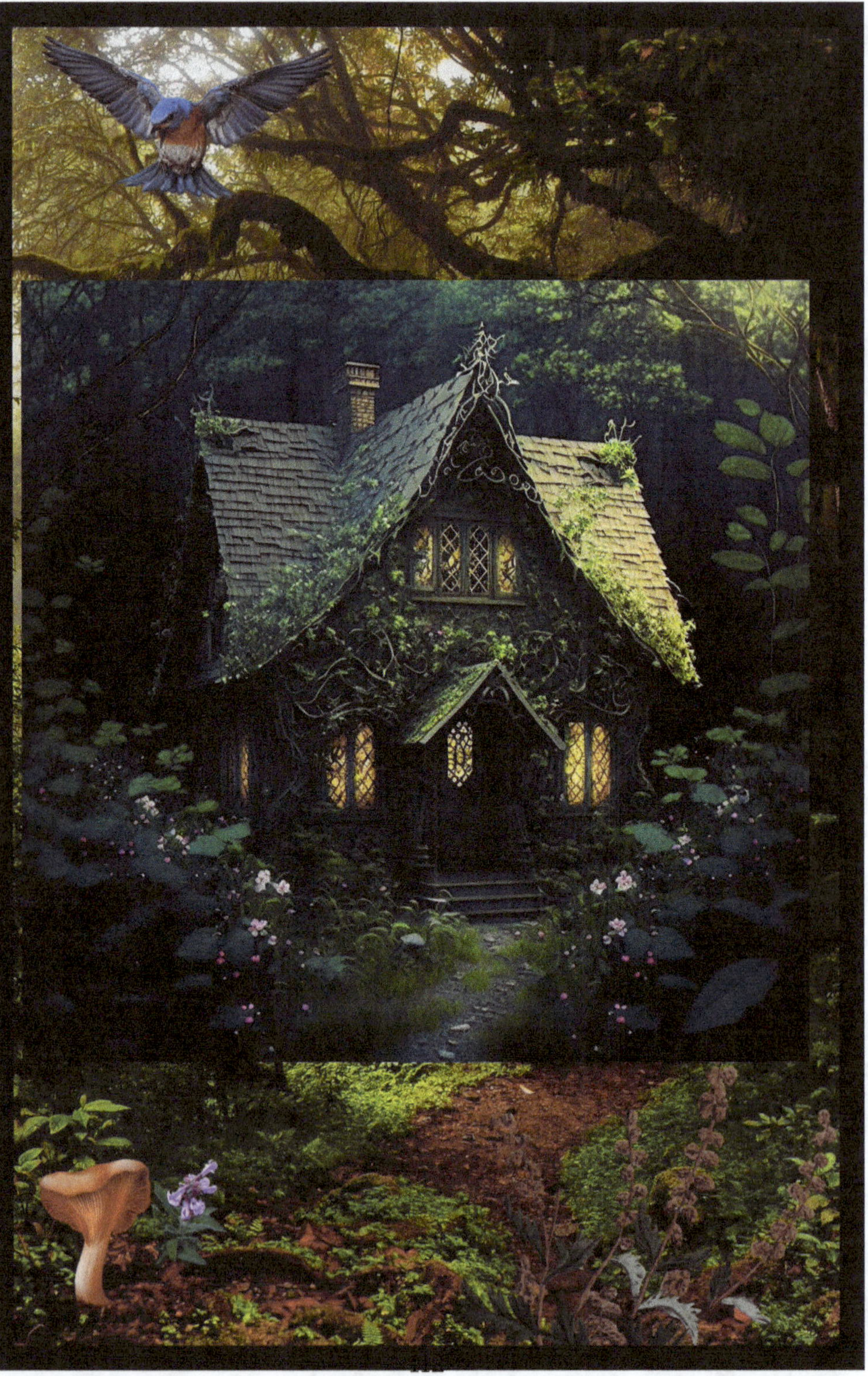

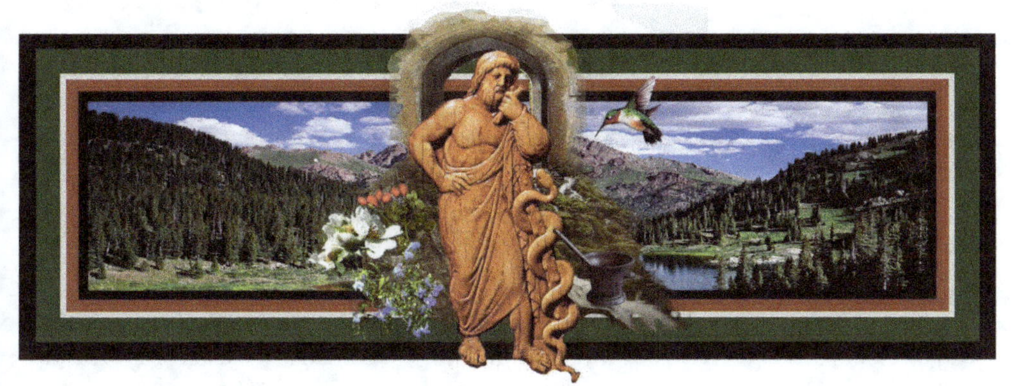

SELF-CARE
FOR THE HEALER
& CARE GIVER

Do you consider yourself a healer or a tender of some kind — perhaps an herbalist or a naturopath, a counselor or therapist, a steward of the land, a justice minded activist, or a family *care-giver*? If so, then you may find you can do the most good when you first *care* about and *give* to yourself.

When we work regular rote jobs just for needed money, we might not care too much about either the work we do or the results down the line. But by its very nature, the work of any kind of healer affects us greatly, on a physical and psychological level. We expend not only time and energy but emotional capital into the people, ecosystems, cultures and societies that seek to aid and mend.

The more that we care, the more personal investment we have in the outcomes.

This depth of caring can mean that we put more effort into our actions, from consultations and assessments to formulations and followups. This means being easier trusted and relied upon by those we try to help, more effective in our wide ranging kinds of efforts to help and to heal, repair and remake — but it also often means that we're daily trying harder, feeling more as well as doing more, and in the throes of our passion and mission we may not even notice the ways in which we're impacted or depleted.

These can manifest as accumulative exhaustion from reduced hours of sleep and hyperactivity, leaving our minds a little less clear and functional. Or as stress, that can slowly damage our immune systems as well as our psychological wellbeing. Or result in our being traumatized ourselves by the traumas of the distraught people we work to help. Or a sneaky buildup of depression, from feeling that we've failed to do enough to resolve a client's or a family member's or even a society's painful conditions.

If you also strongly care about things like healthcare accessibility for the impoverished or marginalized, or about preserving the rights and traditions of natural healing practices in the face of their denigration and regulation, just might may find that you're putting in extra hours every day to provide free or discounted services to the needy, or that you're sometimes confronting official and political systems at the same time. Because we are aware of so much and love so much, it can start feeling like it's our personal, individual responsibility to somehow, some way, fix the whole damn world.

Making the world a better, more healed and whole place does not all fall just on our shoulders, of course, but subconsciously it can feel that way, so much so that nothing we do may feel quite enough. We can get caught up in a loop of constant acceleration as we chase the healer's holy grail, the resolution of dis-ease of all kinds and an end to suffering. And moving so fast, with our eyes so tightly fixed on our goals, it becomes all too easy to neglect our personal needs, ignore our discomforts, and drain our crucial reserves.

At some point it becomes counterproductive, when we eventually get too busy to tend all our clients, tend our important projects, and tend to the home, hobbies and relationships that nourish us. Regardless of how motivated or energetic we are, it's only a matter of time before we become too tired to do our very best thinking. Daily trying to educate, support and cheer up people who are going through difficult periods, leaves us with little capacity for elation and celebration once we quit for the night.

I get the urgency that you feel, with so much illness and injustice to address, and with so much good that you want to give. You have a long to-do list for sure, but you will be way more effective, and be able to serve your mission and aims for many more years, if you put your own bodily, psychological and spiritual needs near the top!

Let's throw out just a few examples for consideration and inspiration:

Make sure you get enough sleep every night, to avoid accumulated sleep debt. A big help is setting aside an hour offscreen, relaxing or playing, right before bed. And you know there are herbal aids from nervines to sleep inducers, and Cannabis tincture can keep you in dreamland better than any pharma products on the shelves.

Eat enough, eat healthy, and try to eat your meals at approximately the same time each day. Pay attention to what you are and aren't ingesting, as well as to what the percentages of nutrients are in each entree. Reduced levels of even a single vitamin such as B-12 or D can have serious ramifications down the line.

Most healing work, other than something like wildland restoration, requires that we be sitting down, and often staring at a computer. The body has to be exercised, challenged, stretched and grown, just as much as the mind does. Step away often, take a break for yoga or workouts, stretch and contort often for at least a minute or two. If you make or dispense herbal medicine, give some your time to sensory stimulating, body utilizing tasks like planting a garden, gathering and wildcrafting.

You give so much to other people, get outside in nature so that the inspirited natural world can give back to you, replenishing your being and spirit. So called forest bathing may be trendy, but it's what humans have done since inception, quieting the mind so as to hear new instructions and lessons, taking into ourselves the energy and affirmation that can come only from the outdoors. Whether in a wild forest, neighborhood park or tiny backyard, it is a vital portal and agent of your revitalization.

Don't forget the importance of both social time and solitude. The interactive company of other people can bolster, stimulate, relax or affirm us. And it is our moments spent all alone, beneath sheltering trees or in a dedicated spot in our rooms, when we can best gather our disparate parts up into a purposed — and refreshed — whole. On that to-do list of yours, make certain to include activities that have little or nothing to do with your work. Following your current interests in unrelated areas can help rewire and refresh your brain, triggering new ways of thinking and perceiving. Even the seemingly most superfluous or indulgent activities are highly valuable, providing not just mental relief but reward.

And follow your bliss. Nah, don't just follow it, do what you have to to live within it, to hold your bliss close even when doing the hardest or most sober of work. Consider what thrilled you most when you were a kid, since those sorts of things would still likely bring you the essential joy. Run barefoot in cool or wet sand, and on pliant grass. Swing from trees. Touch their bark and leaves with eyes closed, so that every shape and texture brings a smile. Rub the sore bodies of loved ones, and allow yourself to be rubbed. Rejoice in your sexuality. Notice the many scents of flowers and the tastes of new foods or of your long valued medicinal potions. Skip, jump, play, sing and dance!

Treat yourself well, and you will find that you're better able to treat unhealthy conditions. Take most excellent care of yourself, and you'll be even more effective at caring for others.

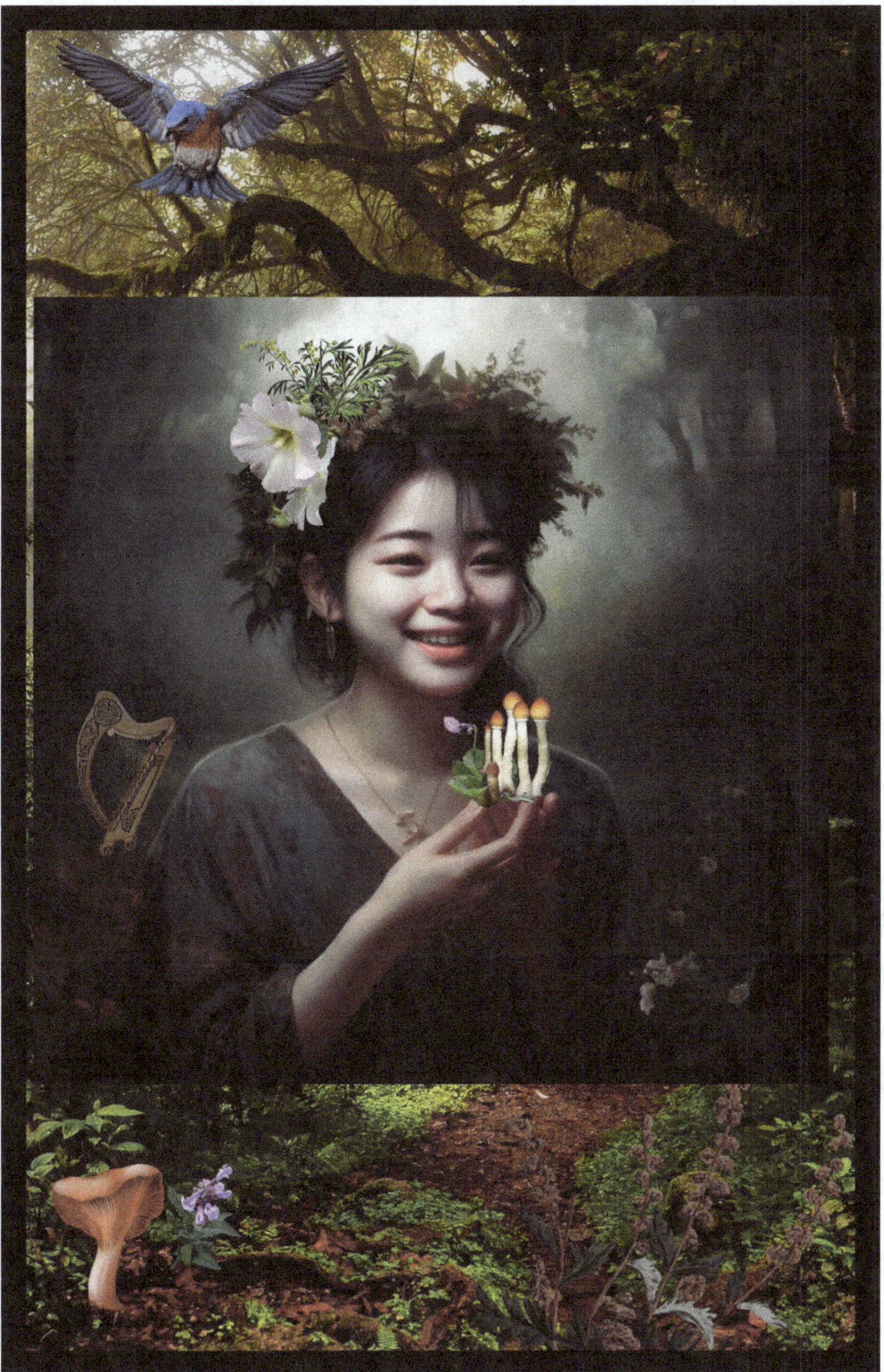

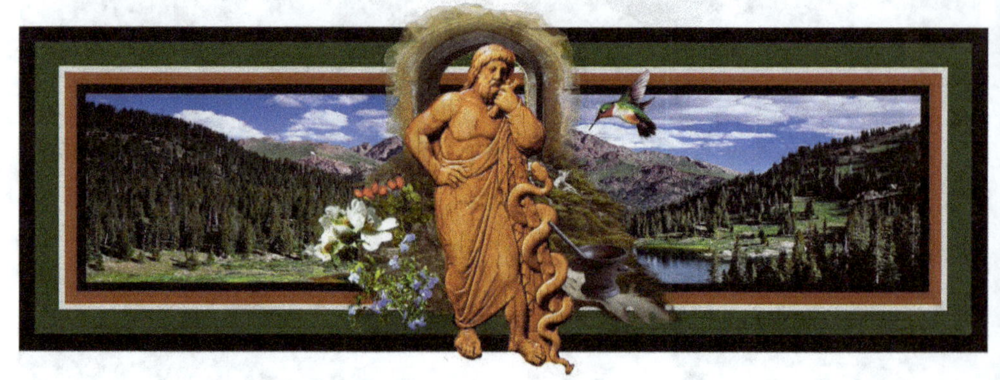

20 QUESTIONS
TO ASK YOURSELF
FOR AN EVEN BETTER HEALER'S LIFE

Imagine your life is a tale that you are the primary creator of — what settings would you like for the backdrops to all you do? As the author, what supportive characters do you want to include in the play that is you? What plot arcs, challenges, redemption, resolution or outcomes?

1. If you knew this was to be your final year of life, what would you do differently? Where would you like to spend your remaining time, with whom? What projects would you give your precious hours to, what experiences would you try to pack in, what guilty pleasures would you want to indulge in and linger with?

2. Likewise, what do you do now, that you'd want to avoid if it was your final year? Would you want to spend your time away from where you live and work now, or apart from the person that you currently live with or the people that you generally work around? Would you really choose to stick to your usual schedule and routines? Would you still be okay with standing in checkout lines, okay with using up hours of your day trying to get somewhere in a car, or with making small talk just to be polite? Would you be as accepting as always of loud unpleasant noises like neighborhood sirens or planes roaring overhead? Would you still feel just as tolerant of bigotry, entitlement, unkindness or injustice?

3. Even if you could be sure of living another hundred years, do you think your life could use a little reappraisal and renovation? What truly serves your health and wholeness, your heart and calling, your aims and dreams, and what do you do or put up with just because it's expected of you? If you were to make a priority list right now of what's most important to you, what things deserve the top spots, and what kinds of stuff might get bumped down closer to the bottom?

4. Who in your life would trigger the greatest pain or longing if they were to move away? What's most important to tell them in person while they're residing close enough to hear?

5. What feels most important for you to always embody?

6. What acts or ways of being do you consider honorable or dishonorable? What do you think of as being your most essential principles, what actions or ways of being do you consider to be inviolable?

7. Under what circumstances does accommodating a person or a protocol actually serve you, and when can it compromise your needs, your ethics or aims?

8. On the other hand, when might your resistance to adjusting and adapting harm you or your hopes?

9. Give it as much thought as needed: What would you say is your overriding, most meaningful purpose on this planet in these times? What can you learn or do to further inspire, empower, equip and energize your purpose?

10. What kind of healer or other practitioner would you most like to be? Do you think you'd be more effective or feel more fulfilled as a community dispenser of herbs and advice, a grower or wildcrafter, a defender of wild habitats, a medicine maker, herb seller, author or teacher? Would it be best for you and your purpose to make a business out of things, or to keep it a passionate interest, a useful hobby, or a free service instead?

11. List all the kinds of the things you'd like to learn if you had the means and time to give.

12. What factors hinder your learning, and what do you have to do to ensure your desired studies and developed understandings?

13. What do you think is most crucial for you to communicate?

14. Do you occasionally get into conflicts without first understanding what the other person is saying, feeling, needing or intending? Do you sometimes get so caught up in thoughts and agendas that you miss out on the messages and colors and scents of the garden or forest you're walking through? Do you ever find yourself eating a meal without hardly noticing the panoply of textures and tastes, or making love with your mind off somewhere else?

15. Take a sensorial inventory of your home, your apothecary and pantry, your yard and you favorite places to walk or gather plants — then consider, which specific sights and sounds and smells would you be saddest to never experience again, and which convey to you the most information and inspiration, which contribute most to your sense of connection or delight?

16. If we think of the world as an organic composition, as an evolving song, then what notes and melodies, inflections and special effects would you like to add?

17. What is your personal definition of "beautiful"? Using your personal metric, what do you find to be beautiful in your world? What can you do to make the things you find less appealing more and more lovely?

18. What might be the biggest ass mistake that you could ever make in your lifetime… and what do you need to do to make sure that never happens?

19. What's the most useful or precious thing that anyone could ever give you? Once you've got a clear picture of what that would be, question if it's something that you can *give to yourself*.

20. What things in your life bring you great meaning, what things strengthen your vitality, encourage and support your excitement to be alive?

With the above twenty answered, you have in hand the beginnings of a personal yardstick by which you can measure your desires and needs, calibrate your proclivities and preferences, and assess your aspirations, efforts and effects.

Acting on this self-knowledge is never easy, of course, but self inquiry makes it possible for us to prioritize what ideas and activities matter most to us, and possible for us to garner the kinds of positive results that we're intending. Activation is requisite if we're ever to wholly be our authentic selves, or if we're going to accept and enjoy any attendant rewards. Activation is the next step if we're really going to honor, maximize and utilize the finest aspects of what we are and can be. Applying our understandings and evaluations makes it possible for us to avoid at least some of the soul-sapping situations and piss poor decisions in the future. These are just some of the questions that can help us make the most of opportunities and savor the many blessings that come our way, providing ourselves with the gift of a genuinely bettered life.

Bravely ask yourselves, my friends. And then lovingly *do*.

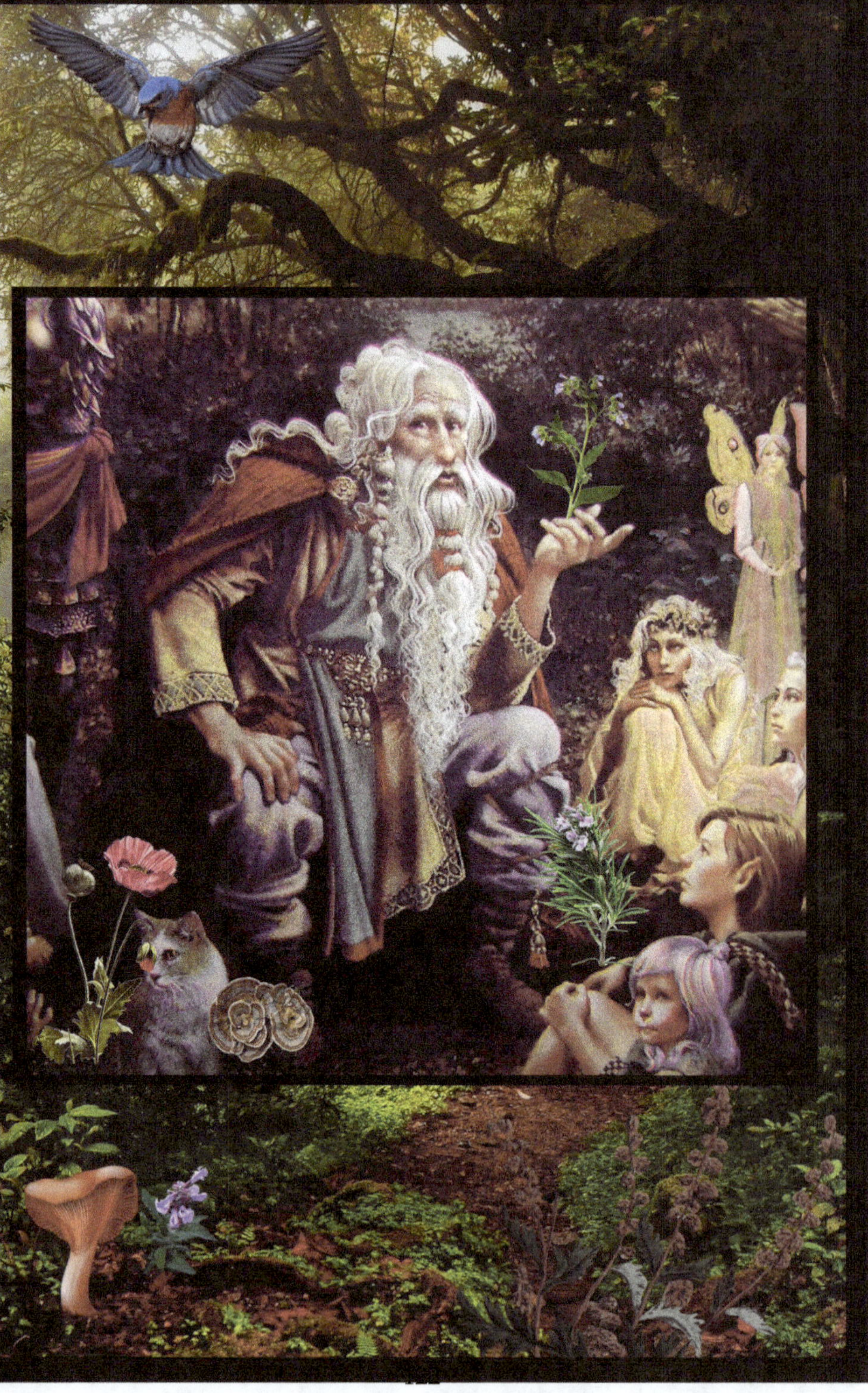

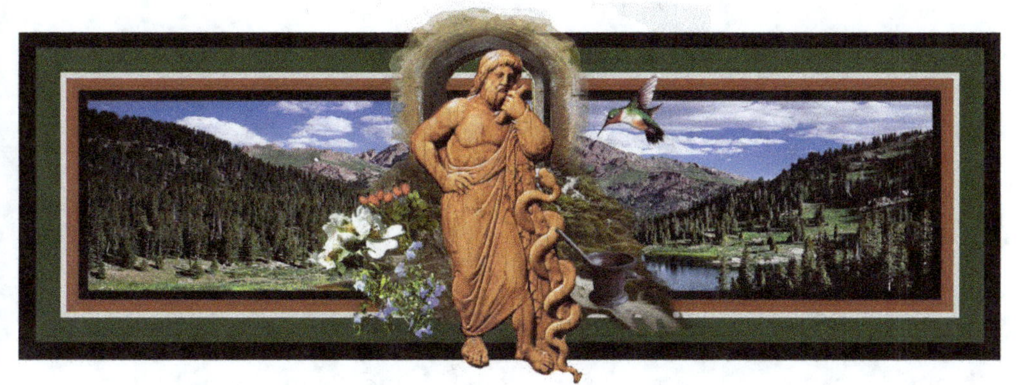

HEALING WORDS
WRITING ABOUT HERBS
& FURTHERING YOUR PERSONAL STORY

From the very first page, the best herbal writings are not only resource and information but a lyrical welcoming – an invitation into a shared state of curiosity and excitement, into the pleasures as well as practicalities of the herbal arts and natural healing.   Whatever our individual needs and educational aims, each time we enter through the words of Plant Healers into a magical commons, a green, vibrant and verdant reality shared by thousands of other plant lovers, medicine makers, nature guardians and culture changers. Every other reader is enjoined with you there, their busy selves barely out of sight on the other side of that emerald grove, wandering through these same forests but on different trails, tending the far end of your garden, learning from the same treasury of shared knowledge, hearing similar calling if from a different muse and set do a different tune, all of us questioning and examining the same Plant Healer's world... from different perspectives, upon this precious common ground.

Words, whether spoken or written, are a gateway to understanding, clarifying for us and equipping us, a transference of what we need to make choices, optimize our offerings, meet our intended goals and fulfill our self assigned purposes. Words can entertain and enliven, enable and empower, fuel and feed. The right strings of words are even a part of how we treat clients and family, in the form of essential explanations, support and

You Too Can Write For Others

You as a reader are not just a recipient, you are an active participant in a dynamic process as you also consider, process, test, extrapolate from, recombine, alter and augment what you read and learn. Then if you distill, summarize, rephrase, and then write down these things, you are indisputably a writer too.

We're all communicants, expressing our thoughts, feelings and wishes through posture, gestures, expressions   and words affecting current happenings and our environs. We all possess some kind and some degree of wisdom that begs to be passed on, we all embody and collect stories that are worth telling. At best, our words suggest the unfolding possibilities of the future, while drawing from and honoring the people, knowings and doings of the past. We give events a life that outlives their participants, and it is called history. We write a letter to our children, and many readings later it becomes an heirloom. We record simple words of gratitude or affection on a napkin from a local bar, and an adoring sweetheart may call it poetry. When we tap away on a computer keyboard, it's based on the conscious or subconscious premise that we have something meaningful to give, and the hope that the reader or listener, the field of natural healing, and perhaps the wider world will somehow be more well and whole as a result. If you've learned anything at all about a subject like herbs, and have any ideas or experiences you can describe, then you too have something worthwhile to share.   You do not need to have practiced natural medicine for decades, some of the best herbalist authors are young or relative newbies but bring fresh and needed new perspectives. The skills required for good writing can be learned by most people, yet no one but you can draw from your own particular set of thoughts, individual experiences, unusual discoveries, ways of looking at and feeling about the world, or intuitive realizations.

Never imagine that writing is only possible for those with the most time on their hands. Quite the contrary. It is the actual doing that gives life to writing, not only the much credited imagination: the physical studying, planting, growing, tasting, pondering, formulating, trying, testing, and dispensing of plant medicines for example. And the false leads and stumbling blocks, misdirection and errors, self satisfying illusions and hope-fed inaccuracies, difficulties and disappointments that lead to more accurate conclusions, more powerful writing, and more helpful treatments.

Plant Healer authors are – without exception – doers, squeezing the hours of writing their magazine articles, blogs and books into days already filled with deadlines and demands, between responsibilities to families and the means of income, teaching classes and traveling, helping out at free community clinics, staffing the first aid tents or administering herbal tonics to the homeless, taking the financial risk of launching new herb stores, making herbal medicines or body care products, or even working a fill time job outside of the herbal field in order to pursue an herbal mission after work, as well as tending or advising nearly everyone who requests it of them. They manage to write in the hours after the children are in bed, or before sunup when the rest of the family arises and needs attention. They write while strapped into their seats thousands of feet in the air, and in airport lounges while waiting to be picked up and driven to the next Good Medicine Confluence they teach at. Some write during boring lectures at college and others between grading the papers of their graduate students, when it's Sunday and everyone else is resting, or while the dinner cooks, noses alert to make sure nothing burns while they weave words on a computer's plastic keys.

Threads spread from writer to reader, and from reader to reader, spreading facts and passions, impetus and vibe like fungal filaments feeding the roots of our enchanted forest and healing traditions.   Every Plant Healer storyteller provides not only the gift of their personal knowledge but of inspiration and instigation, prompting and propelling each listener's explorations and directions, their studies and discoveries, practices and commitments. We are encouraged to add to our own knowledge, further our own skills, deepen our own experiences, and develop our own voices, so that we all can pass our gifts on to others, instructing, and helping.

Effects & Rewards

I've received more than a few emails asking "Why do you give so much to writing?" Tis a couple of reasonable questions, given how much of my finite mortal existence is given to the act of writing for you all, and is especially poignant considering my natural aversion to computers and Luddite abhorrence of plastic, and my constant ache to be outside wandering without a mission along along the wild trails next to Anima Sanctuary's wondrous winding river.

Okay, I'll explain: Writers write to reach outside of of our isolated selves, to maybe touch the hearts of others through the crafted expression of our own experiences, feelings and cares. We write to express ourselves and promote our interests. To provide information that can help other people, and that might even be able to help some folks with their work of aiding others. We write to question authority and resist injustice, to preserve and to celebrate what is truly valuable. We write to educate our allies, entertain our friends and confound our oppressors. We write for kids who are looking for something to believe in, starting with themselves. For our elders, whose adventures and deeds deserve a proper telling. For the plants, who need us to champion them. And for ourselves, to sate this need and fulfill this calling, and to satisfy our hunger to to better the world, to stir, to educate, to express our hearts, to open and to share.

There is income to be made from creating and selling books, writing the narration for videos, or give talks based on our thoughtful wordage, but compensation for the crafting comes in many other ways and forms as well. The act of writing helps us to revisit what we know and have done, develop and refine our thoughts, reassess our conclusions, explore new angles and ramifications, and experiment with how best to present and communicate our ideas. The articles or scripts or posts we make can do double or triple duty as future books or even as course materials if we want to teach. And our writings can bring attention to our gifts, our services, projects and products. Things we write bring attention to all of our offerings, increase the number of students seeking our lessons, result in invites to give presentations or participate in other productions, and lead to greater sales of the medicines and other things we might make.

Foremost among the rewards, however, is simply the satisfaction that comes from giving voice to who we are and what we feel, sharing what one has to offer, making a unique difference in people's lives and in this way fulfilling a long held dream and evolving purpose. Writers certainly need to "make a living," but the magic of our craft is how it can contribute to our making a life for ourself and benefit the lives of others. What we seek more than to make money, make medicines or make new books, is to make a difference – a difference in folks' health and how they approach healing, in the perceptions and values of the society and communities we are enmeshed in, in the ways that people treat each other, the land, and our kindred species.

That's not to say that writing or teaching is easy, not even for the most gifted. In spite of all the talking that our species does, communicating clearly and fully is getting increasingly rare and never hugely easy. Our species is increasingly handicapped by shortening attention spans, and trained to reduce or abbreviate by all the phone texting we do and the various online platforms that limit the number of characters in a message.

Communication is a craft that is best in longer packets of information and thought, dressed in evocative and even lovely phrasing. It is preceded by conscious unhurried consideration, determined and sorted according to its relevance and our intent, with the potential effects of all the possible words on the targeted audiences. We necessarily write in styles that different kinds of readers can "hear," relate to and be affected by. Poetic expression is as ill suited to academic and "professional" periodicals and publishers as is an academic style a poor approach when trying to reach, entice, equip or enrich newbies, generalists and laymen. Our Plant Healer publications have been a blend of the latest research and traditional folklore, ever reexamined scientific evidence and subjective personal experiences, plant mythology and materia medica means that we feature articles and quarterly columns that integrate all of these and more. We ask our writers to speak authentically in their own individual voices, from their exerience and training, but also from their hearts – that they speak their passions, that their words are lit up by their excitement about each plant or topic.

As someone who edits as well as composes, I can offer you at least a few practical suggestions:

- Determine what information, discoveries, techniques, experiences, lessons and messages you are most able and enthused to impart.

- Be sure to study ahead of time the submission guidelines of the magazine, book publisher, or self publishing service – including total words length and formatting requirements.

- Tighten the focus for each article section or book chapter, avoiding non-sequiturs and digressions.

- Determine your primary audience, the needs and proclivities you will want to address, and the vernacular, aesthetic and writing style that will be most effective for the various kinds of readers.

- Start every article or chapter with an introductory paragraph that delineates the topic and hints at the overall lesson or conclusion, that paints a picture, that sets things in a physical place that can evoke and engage a reader's physical senses, that establishes a mood, and that awakens reader interest and curiosity.

- Determine what is most crucial to present and vital to the point or theme.

- Organize these elements in a way that readily makes sense, with each paragraph proceeding from the foundations and tenets of those which come before.

- Extrapolation and leaps of thought are great, if grounded in what you know. Beware of repeating even the most common "facts" unless you have tested them in practice or experienced them yourself.

- Cite your thinking and evidence leading to any conclusions or recommendations.

- Consider creating a balance of conceptual and practical elements, the whys as well as hows.

- Consider connecting thoughts and expositions to functions, actions and applications.

- Quote sources rather than paraphrasing them, and provide attribution.

- End articles and chapters with a conclusion, and perhaps relate it topically and tonally to the writing's introduction.

- Leave the reader with a literal sense of what you are sharing, with a feeling and motivation, as well as with facts and means that they can utilize.

Plant Healer writers are artists ever working to improve their art, presenting dependable information of importance to people's health, rooted in the history of our field, responding to the call and needs of the coming generations, and told through the stories of each writer's evolving lives.

Good writing is informed and colored by real life happenings, heartened by human emotions and sensations, and this is as true for the writings of herbalists as it is for the crafters of fine fiction.

Your Life as a Story You Create

Story is at the very heart of human existence, defining, communicating and preserving cumulative experience, meaning and lesson. Stories are some of the most effective ways that we people have ever made sense of ourselves and our world. Story provides us a framework for our identity, expresses our interests, hopes and fears, and defines our personal roles... fueling motivation, providing direction and making manifestation possible. Telling stories is as elemental as breathing and even more definitively human, for while breathing keeps us alive, it is the richness and significance of our story that can make our finite existence feel truly worth living and sharing.

The problem comes when we think of ourselves as mere characters in stories that other people, groups and power elites are the authors of. The individual and collective struggles are real, and the controls and influences of the dominant paradigm are ominous, but we need not leave it to anyone else to define, limit, or impart meaning to our experiences, any more than to determine our truths, path and direction. It is up to us to each recast ourselves and our stories in the light of what is most significant to us, our self image, our work and play. How we most like to envision ourselves and our long plot arc, can indeed be the tale we increasingly embody, fulfill, and take great pleasure in.

In addition, our most personal story is a significant element in the ongoing tales of folk herbalism. We are each both the central character in the book of our unfolding existence, and one of the most influential authors and determinants of our personal life and practice. With each word we send out into the world, we can help to collectively determine the shapes and flavors, power and direction of herbalism today and in the future.

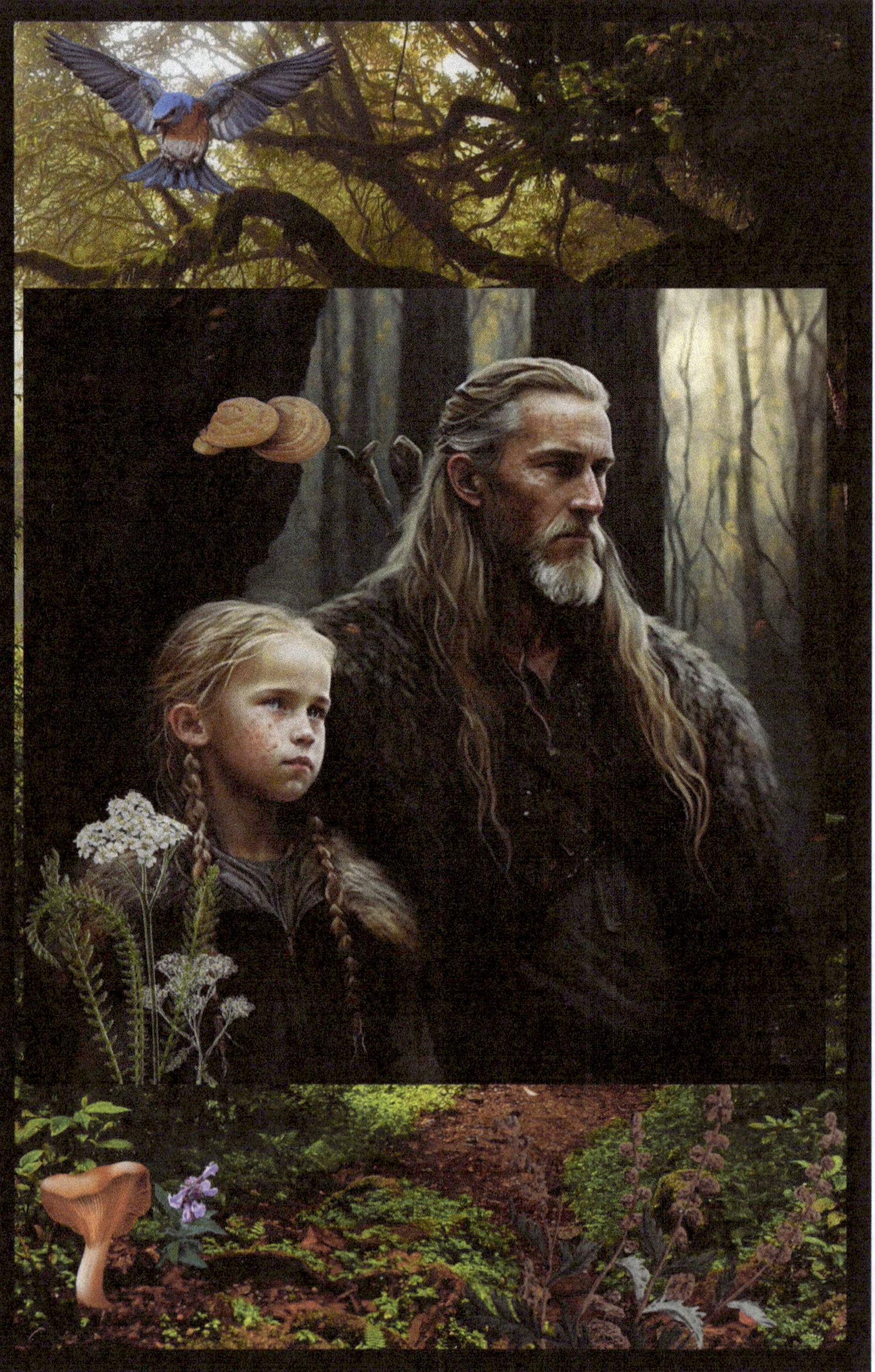

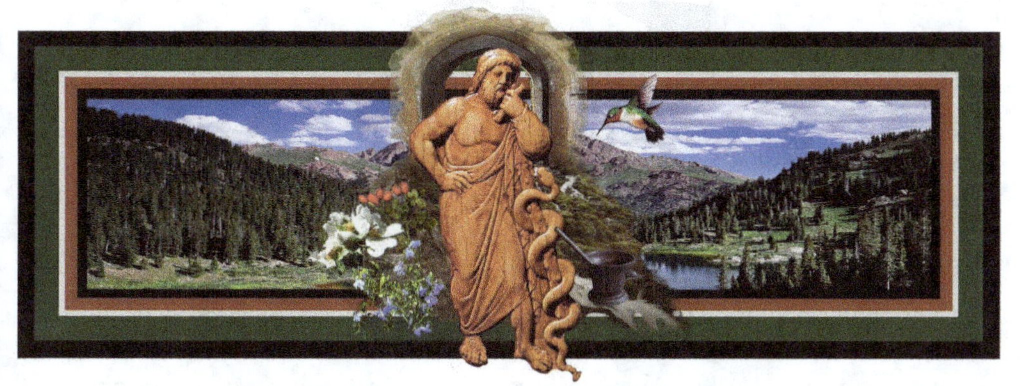

GROWING OUR FUTURES

TAKING RESPONSIBILITY FOR WHAT WE PLANT OR PROPAGATE, TEND OR NEGLECT IN LIFE

"There's nothing we can do about the greater course of things" I've been told, but that's only partly true. Politicians will remain lame no matter how we vote, the big-money interests will continue making the rules. On the other hand, how we respond can affect what happens, in small ways often, and other times in ways that are revolutionary and paradigm shattering. Rather than fearing what seems like an ever degrading future, we can see what part we play in unfolding events, and play it better. We can see how our ignorance, imagined powerlessness and ignoble acceptance actually enables the oppression, greed and insanity of the power-brokers, and we can act deliberately to determine what proceeds from our toiling or avoiding, passive ignoring or active *tilling*.

Tilling, he said, as the source of the noun "future" is very much a plant related one. Its "root" is the ancient IndoEuropean verb "to grow," as in helping to grow a life sustaining home garden or essential village crop... or in the days before agriculture, assisting the proliferation of wild, edible and medicinal plants upon which they depended. Note that I said "verb," the reality of the future appearing to even paleolithic people as an obvious product of not only circumstance and supernatural or divine forces, but of their own actions as well, determined by a person's values and needs, oriented in the direction of a vision, focused on an effect or outcome.

The future, therefore, is not a state but a process, not a predetermined destination but an unfolding, an action. It is a "doing," and in part it is *our* doing, a product of how we live our lives, and of a mixture of the both beneficial and unhealthy, wise and unwise choices that we make. We may make this contribution largely unconsciously, blaming our woes on unfair God or circumstances we consider outside our control, or else on those abusive mates, oppressive agencies or supposed authorities that we imagine have power over us as helpless victims. Or alternatively, we can become aware of how we affect and alter the world, of the ways in which we contribute to the endless chain of cause and effect, with our future and that of our communities and our land becoming an increasingly deliberate, attentive, caring, purposeful and will-driven result of our well meaning intention and resolute efforts.

The future is in a sense unavoidable, and yet its form is neither inevitable, irreversible nor unalterable. It is our personal responsibility – our individual and collective ability-to-respond — that to some degree determines the shape and degree of the tragedy and loss, lessons and benefits that are to come. It is not something to explain away, default on, submit to or cope with... but rather, it's more like something that we help to make and grow, that we disseminate and plant the seeds of, then either tend and nourish or neglect and thus imperil or strengthen. We each help co-create what sprouts and flourishes, the ways that it branches and spreads, as well as helping determine creates an imbalance in its ecosystem, visibly suffers or prematurely dies. Whether we are aware of our role or not, we have a hand in what we harvest and ingest, what we painfully bear or are excitedly rewarded with. Future results, events and situations, gifts and effects arise not not so much as undeserved blessings, and certainly not as penalty or curse, but as the vegetal-like "produce" of what we do and don't do, and optimally a reflection of our awakened and directed efforts.

The future is not our crop, but it is to whatever degree an outgrowth of what we do and don't do. It's what will manifest whether we notice or understand it, own up to our part in its creation or defer the responsibility. But in the root sense of the word, it is also what we as reality-gardeners grow. Growing our awareness and knowledge, sensory awakeness and awakened instincts and intuition. Our health and wholeness, our abilities, effectiveness and repertoire of skills. Our children. Our marriages and other relationships. Our homes. Our books, paintings, projects and missions. Our gardens of sustenance and plant-inspired delight. Our loves and lives.

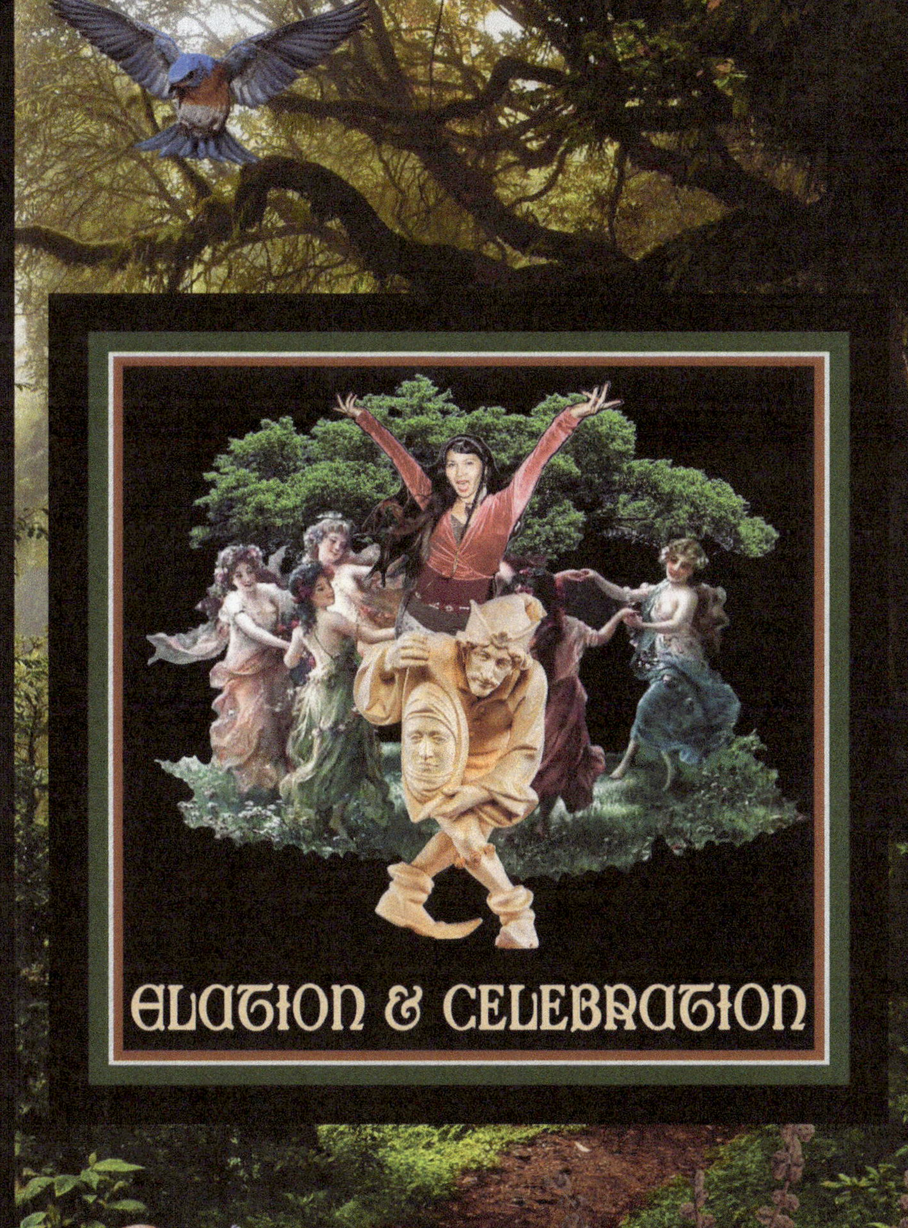

ELATION & CELEBRATION

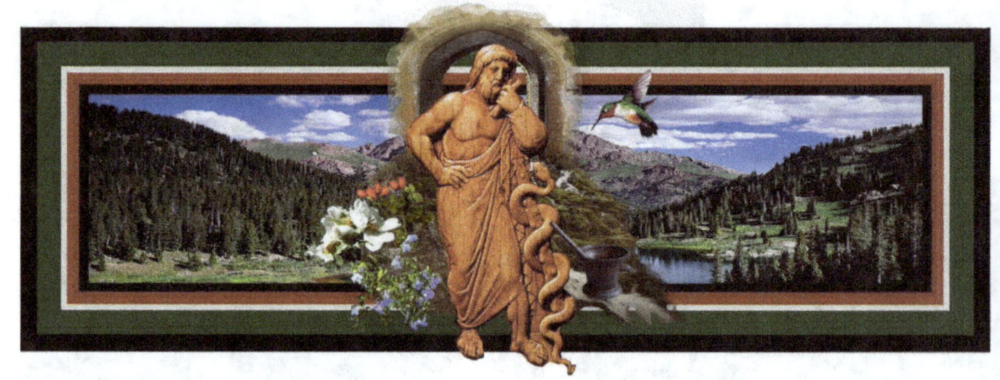

THE RESILIENT HEALER
TRYING TIMES, INFINITE POSSIBILITIES, & WILD CELEBRATION

Herbalists, healers and culture-shifters of all stripes face trying times, times of corporate hegemony and social conformity, environmental destruction and injustice, widespread resignation and crippling complacency. We're in a crucial period when we need to act to ensure herbal access and justice, and have to do a lot more to protect the plants that heal and inform us. But we're also living in a place and time of infinite possibilities, of more choices than ever before, and with potentially more information, greater synthesis and deeper comprehension, as well as stronger motivations to take action and follow our paths.

In spite of all the challenges, obstacles and handicaps, it remains possible to better orient ourselves in the physical world, and to explore our personal gifts, needs, feelings, purpose and direction. It remains possible to deepen our awareness and understanding of natural authentic self. Possible to awaken our bodily senses, learning to better sense the world we are an integral part of. To recognize more patterns and notice more beauty, to hear more exquisitely, to taste every nuance of our food, to savor even the mundane details of our mortal lives. To tap our bodily knowing and creature instincts, and sometimes to increase intuition. To deepen our sense of place... of family, home, land, ecosystem and bioregion. It's still possible to further our awareness of and active relationship to the natural, revelatory world.

It's in our power to recognize the intrinsic nature of and animating force in everything, and every thing's intrinsic value apart from human use. To increase our sense of self worth and confidence, based on our true abilities rather than imposed or imagined characteristics and gifts. To come to better understand our fears, and how to use our fears as markers for what needs our attention, as fuel to act, as motivation to change what needs changing. To realize that we are a co-creators of not only our reality but our world, and commit to acting accordingly. To discover how to give back to the earth that provides and inspires. It remains possible to learn how to grow from our every mistake and misdirection. To get beyond victimhood. To detach from unhealthy habits, expectations, judgments, and ways of thinking. To develop healthy attachments to life, spirit, values and missions. To make every moment a decisive moment, and take responsibility for both what we do and what we don't do. To reawaken a childlike sense of wonder and connection. To learn how to best utilize our gifts and skills for the good of ourselves and the world. It's still possible to discover how we can actively fulfill our individual most meaningful purposes. And to learn to better celebrate and deeper savor!

The need and calling for self-care and community care skills like herbalism has never been greater. As the price of pharmaceuticals continually goes up and their dangers become ever more evident, and whenever the general economy is shaky, herbal knowledge is again accepted as it was in the days before the advent of "modern" medicine — as essential. There is a new and rising wave of herbalists of all ages, insistent on learning the old ways and the new twists, treating their families or serving their communities. It's that which has us giving nearly all of my time to these projects, and the satisfaction that comes with helping to feed and further this aroused herbal renaissance.

Empowered folk herbalism is only one piece — albeit an important one — in what is a larger interweaving of social action, earth stewardship and crucial cultural change. With increased attention to the self-empowering field of plant medicine, we will again and again be making the connection to the necessary, active healing of our wounded hearts and psyches, healing the schism between us and the rest of nature, healing our communities and the damaged earth that we and our herbs together grow from. Trying times be damned. Dire circumstances and immense challenges are part of what makes this most vital work not just important, but a true cause for our wild celebration!

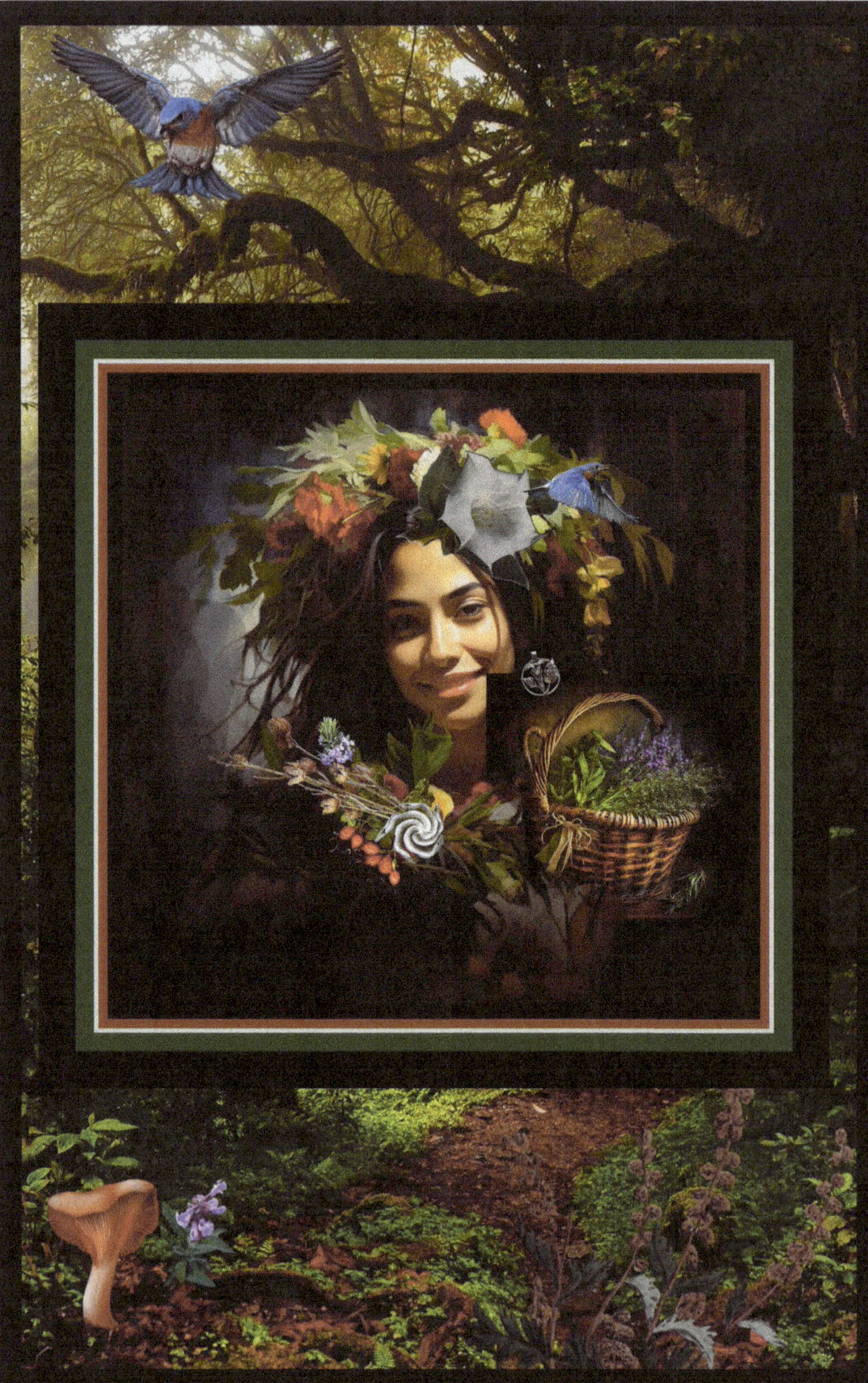

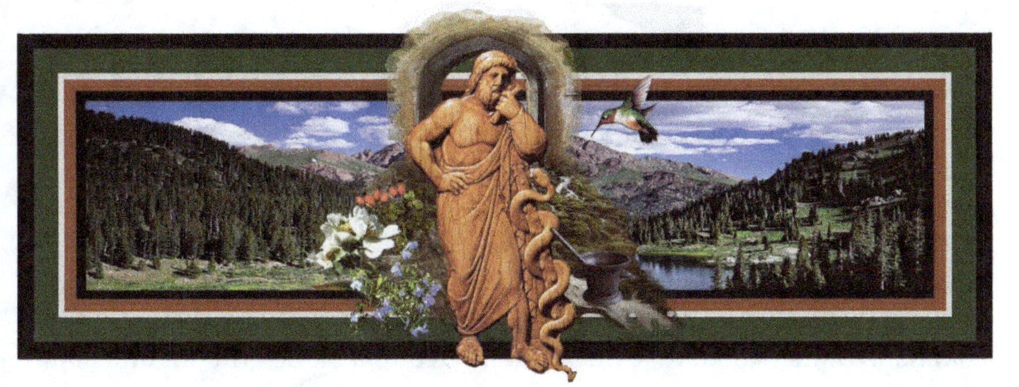

YOUR MISSION
RIDING THE PASSIONS
OF PURPOSE

Many of you have what feels like a mission to you, a lifelong purpose and goal centered around what feels most significant, most needed, and most satisfying. This is fortunately sometimes the same as our career, but it can also be what we care about so much that we give the majority of our free time to it.

Most of my readers are herbalists, culture shifters and healers of one kind or another. You may have found a way to make your living from making and selling tinctures, or seeing and helping clients, or even leading classes for eager students. Or you may be funding your herbal work and interests with a regular job, subsidizing what you love by doing things you have to. Or maybe you are a homemaker or homesteader, with a mission to take care of the health needs of your family, neighborhood or region. Either way, healing and plants have probably come to feel central to who you are and to what you feel born and meant to do.

One thing's for sure, you mission is never simply doing what you think is most needed, nor just what gets the most approval, or what makes you the most money. Neither is it simply doing something we enjoy, even though one indication that we're on a mission is how incredibly compelling, gratifying and satisfying we find even the most arduous and challenging aspects of our work.

It is our personal mission that determines the optimum role that we — our natures, our constitutions, characteristics, abilities, predilections and interests – can admirably fill in our lives. Having a known mission can be one of the greatest gifts we ever receive, while also being one of the most significant of services that we could ever give.

I have a sense that we — as integral elements, agents and organs of the planetary whole – are informed by that whole at a deeper level than commonly understood, that we are connected to a biotic grid not unlike the way trees are hooked up to and can communicate through a vast fungal mat just beneath the ground to an energetic network that connects all things, and through which the whole exerts influences on the direction of its parts. If so, a tailored mission may be the way in which we are best purposed. And if so, it's something that we certainly need to recognize, choose, assume, and determinedly act on. In no sense is a mission an assignment from some external authority, it's a self identified cause whose aims and ways we give our all too. It's nothing like a fate that we've got little say in, but more like a purposed destiny that we must first recognize and then embrace, a very personal path that we feel both called and equipped to take.

No matter how we identify, whether it be Plant Healers or medicine makers, artists or musicians, hands-on parents or dedicated teachers, spiritual leaders or culture-rocking visionaries, social activists or the restorers and nurturers of the land — our mission is our *passion*, and enlivened and fulfilled are we who ride our passions like dragons in a well chosen direction… a mission that in its own special way contributes simultaneously to both our own actualization and the healing and wholeness of the world.

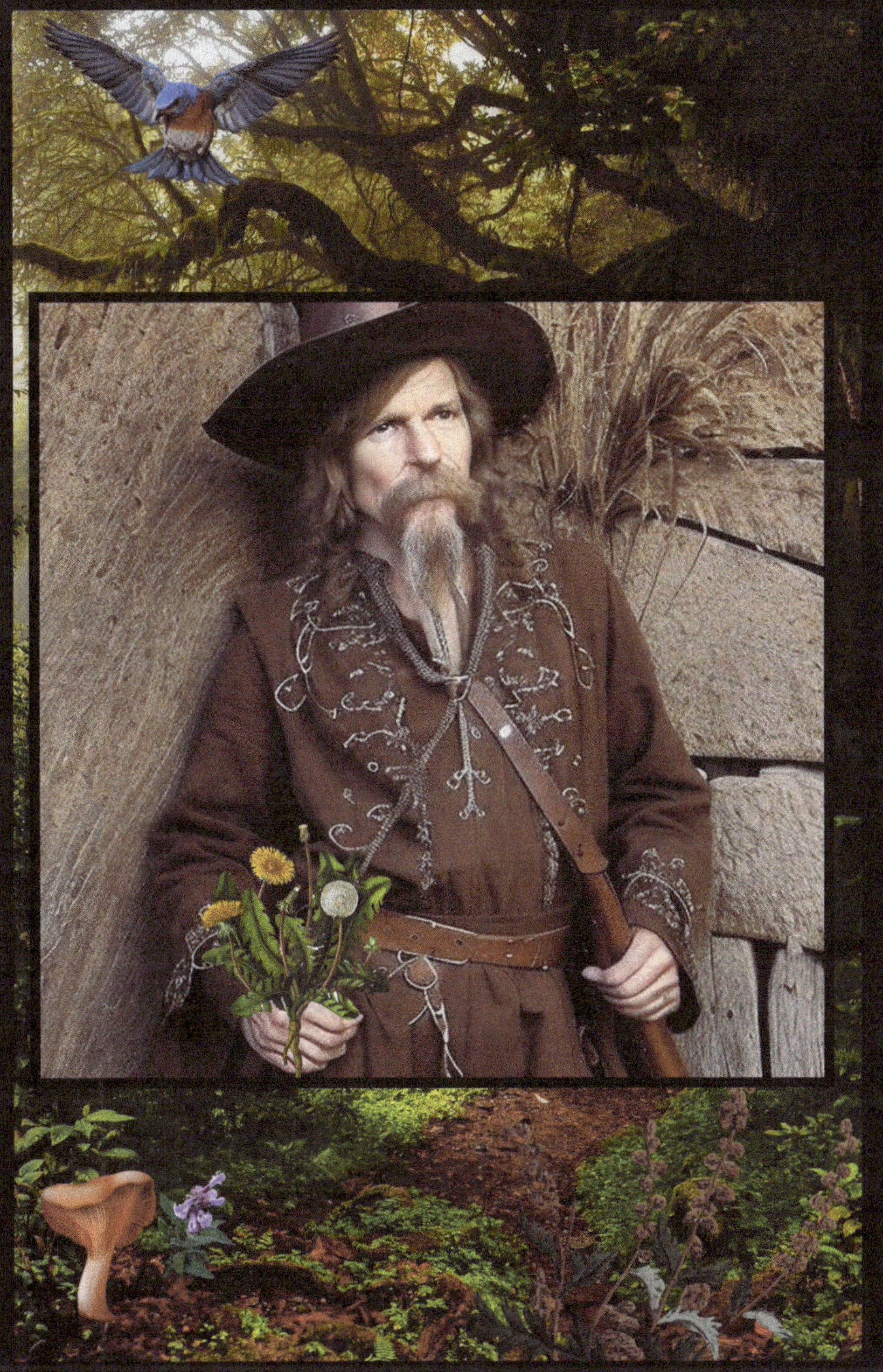

Jesse Wolf Hardin is an impactful author, ecosopher, ecological and societal activist, personal counsel, graphic artist, musician, historian, and grateful father — a champion of both human and bio diversity as well as of nature's medicines. Wolf has been a featured presenter at hundreds of conferences and universities, and was the creator of cross cultural ecospiritual collaborations appropriately called "Medicine Shows" that melded his spoken word with live music, indigenous presenters, and focused activism. In 2008 he cofounded with Kiva Rosethorn the international Good Medicine Confluence gathering, along with the in-depth digital magazine for herbalists, healers and folklorists *Plant Healer Quarterly* (available at: www.PlantHealerMagazine.com) Wolf is also the cocreator of the *Hedge Guild Oracle* deck and book featuring his artwork, bringing clarity to our self exploration and daily options and choices. He has had over 800 articles appear in over 200 different publications, and is the author of over 25 books including early titles like *Full Circle, Kindred Spirit* and *Gaia Eros,* along with *The Practice of Herbalism* and *The Plant Healer's Path* covering the core whys and hows of an herbal practice, *The Healing Terrain* on sense of place, wildcrafting and cultivation, and the healing powers of nature, as well as an historical novel *The Medicine Bear,* a book of herbs and empowerment for children *I'm a Medicine Woman Too!* (Hops Press 2009), and *The Traveling Medicine Show: Pitchmen & Plant Healers of Early America.* His book *The Enchanted Healer* explores expanded awareness, heightened senses, the spirit and magic of plants, and personal reenchantment, while his latest writings can be found in *The Herbalist: Your Healer's Journey.* You can purchase most of his books as well as the Oracle set at PlantHealerBookstore.com, and watch at no cost Wolf's inspirational Plant Healer Path video series at YouTube.com/ @HerbRally. Check the full range of Plant Healer offerings and subscribe to the free and informative *Herbaria Monthly* zine at: PlantHealer.org

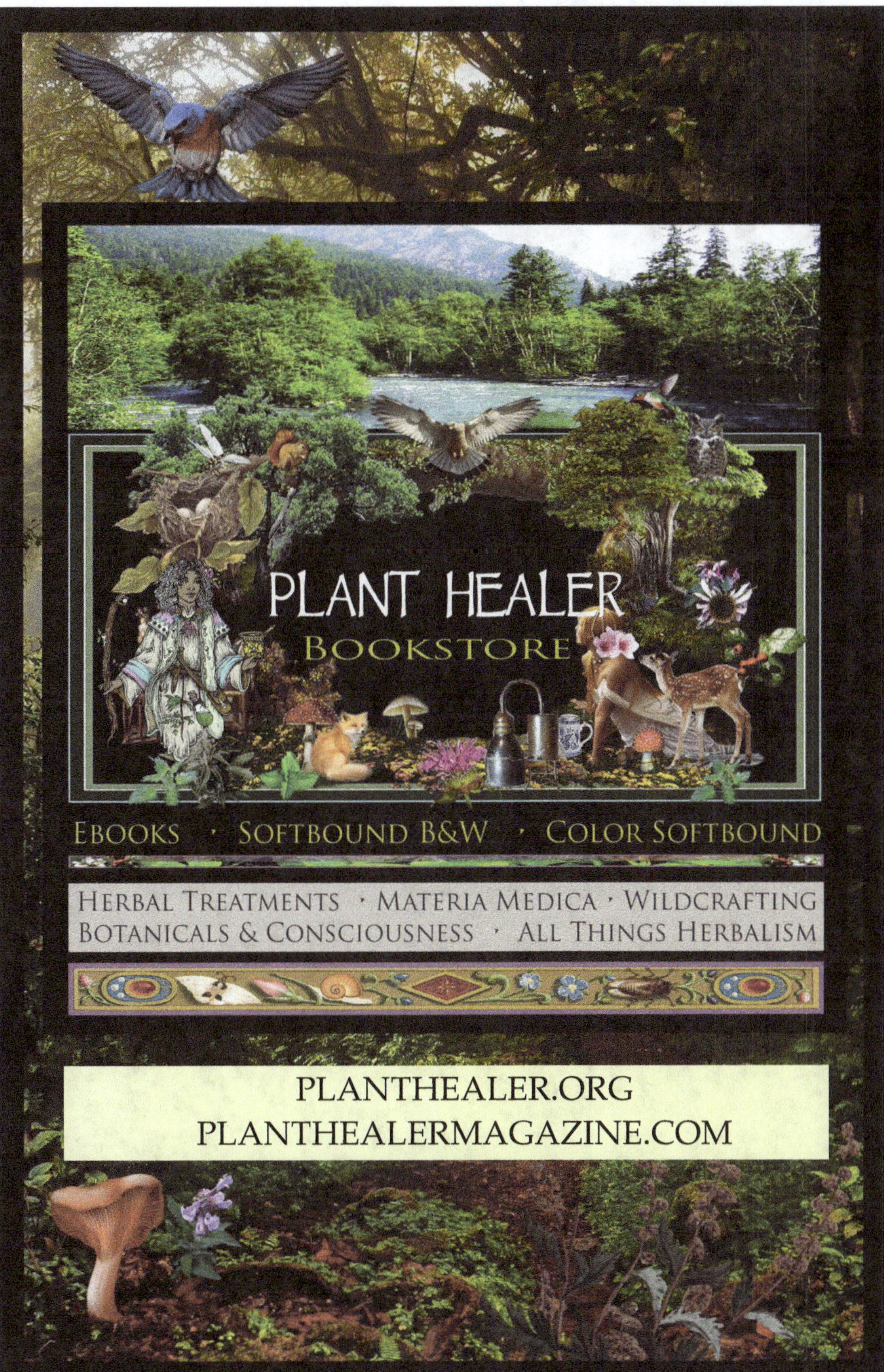

PLANT HEALER
BOOKSTORE

EBOOKS · SOFTBOUND B&W · COLOR SOFTBOUND

HERBAL TREATMENTS · MATERIA MEDICA · WILDCRAFTING
BOTANICALS & CONSCIOUSNESS · ALL THINGS HERBALISM

PLANTHEALER.ORG
PLANTHEALERMAGAZINE.COM

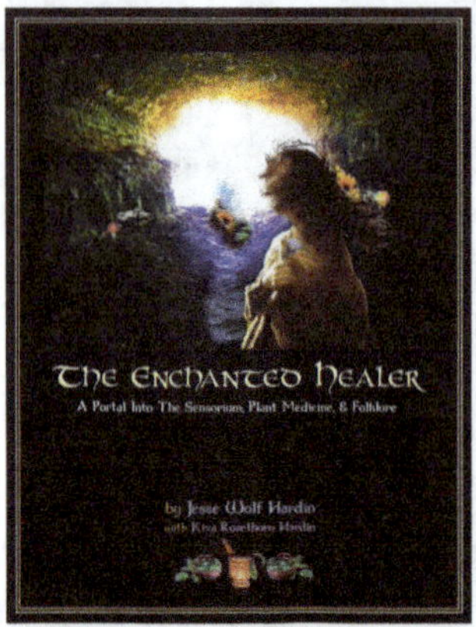

THE ENCHANTED HEALER
A Portal Into The Sensorium, Plant Medicine, & Folklore
by Jesse Wolf Hardin
with Kiva Rosethorn Hardin

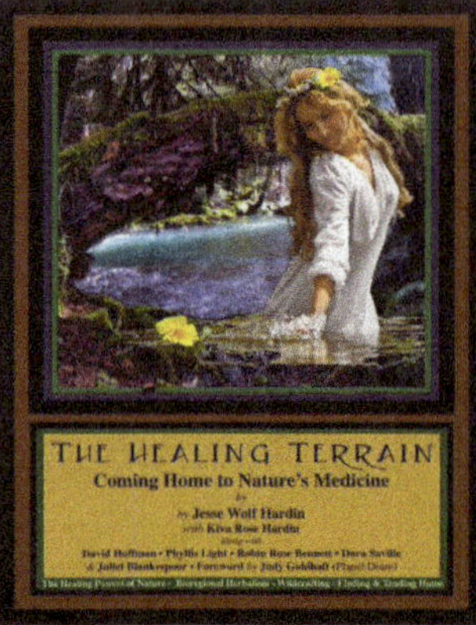

THE HEALING TERRAIN
Coming Home to Nature's Medicine
by Jesse Wolf Hardin
with Kiva Rose Hardin

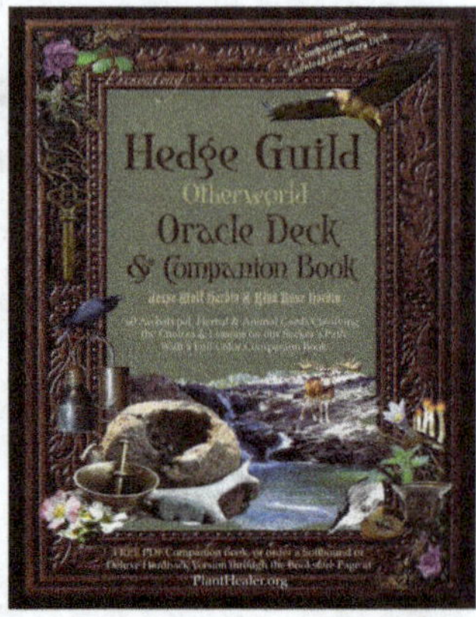

Hedge Guild
Otherworld
Oracle Deck
& Companion Book
Jesse Wolf Hardin & Kiva Rose Hardin
PlantHealer.org

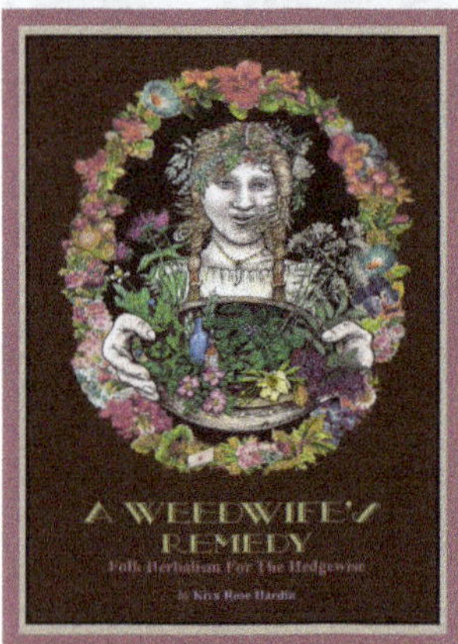

A WEEDWIFE'S
REMEDY
Folk Herbalism For The Hedgewise
by Kiva Rose Hardin

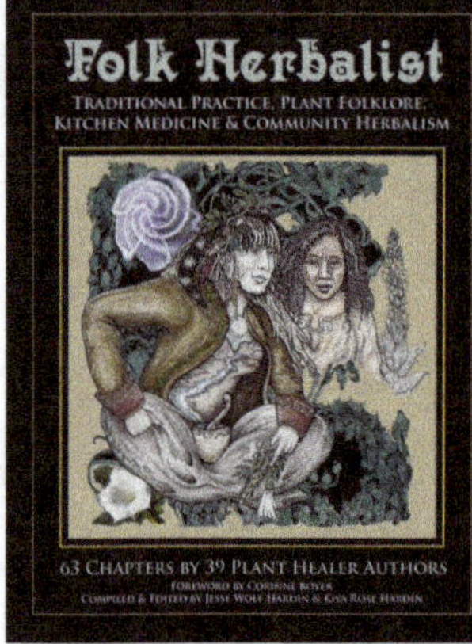

Folk Herbalist
TRADITIONAL PRACTICE, PLANT FOLKLORE,
KITCHEN MEDICINE & COMMUNITY HERBALISM
63 CHAPTERS BY 39 PLANT HEALER AUTHORS
FOREWORD BY CORINNE BOYER
COMPILED & EDITED BY JESSE WOLF HARDIN & KIVA ROSE HARDIN

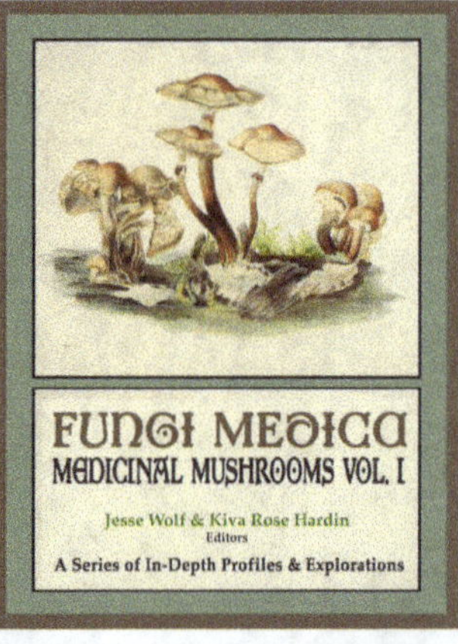

FUNGI MEDICA
MEDICINAL MUSHROOMS VOL. I
Jesse Wolf & Kiva Rose Hardin
Editors
A Series of In-Depth Profiles & Explorations

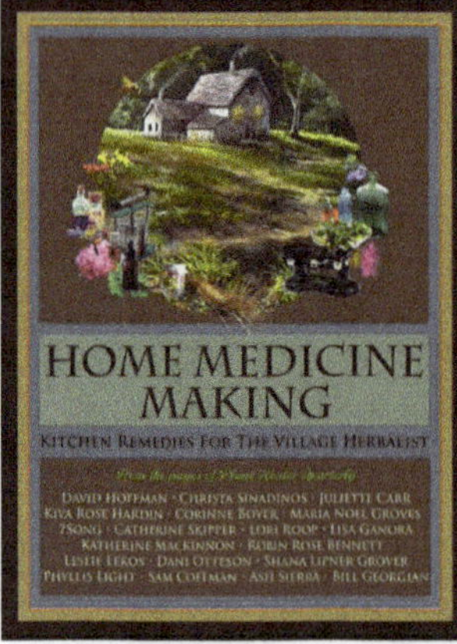

HOME MEDICINE
MAKING
KITCHEN REMEDIES FOR THE VILLAGE HERBALIST
DAVID HOFFMAN · CHRISTA SINADINOS · JULIETTE CARR
KIVA ROSE HARDIN · CORINNE BOYER · MARIA NOEL GROVES
7SONG · CATHERINE SKIPPER · LORI ROOP · LISA GANORA
KATHERINE MACKINNON · ROBIN ROSE BENNETT
LESLIE LEKOS · DANI OTTESON · SHANA LIPNER GROVER
PHYLLIS LIGHT · SAM COFFMAN · ASH SIERRA · BILL GEORGIAN

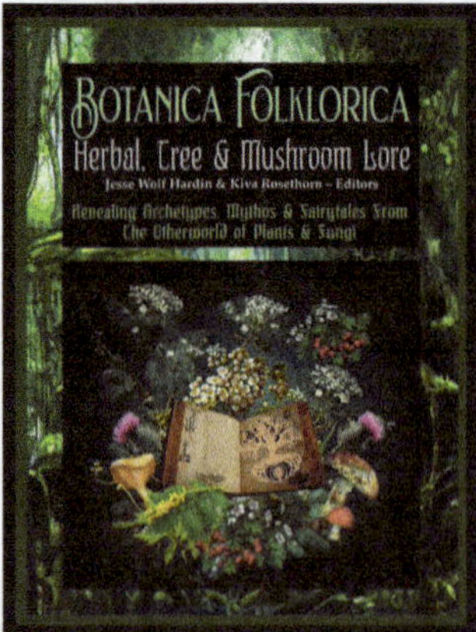

BOTANICA FOLKLORICA
Herbal, Tree & Mushroom Lore
Jesse Wolf Hardin & Kiva Rosethorn - Editors
Revealing Archetypes, Mythos & Fairytales from
The Otherworld of Plants & Fungi

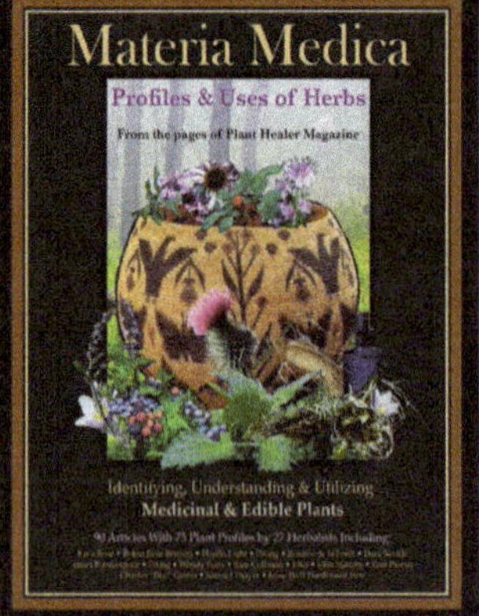

Materia Medica
Profiles & Uses of Herbs
From the pages of Plant Healer Magazine
Identifying, Understanding & Utilizing
Medicinal & Edible Plants

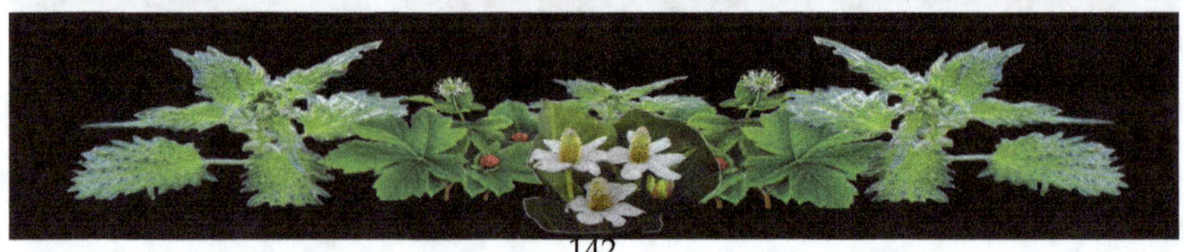